Jewish American Parents Navigating Autism Supports

Beth L. Raiola

Jewish American Parents Navigating Autism Supports

Exploring Culturally Responsive Services, Advocacy, and Schooling

palgrave
macmillan

Beth L. Raiola
Davie, FL, USA

ISBN 978-3-032-29298-8 ISBN 978-3-032-29299-5 (eBook)
https://doi.org/10.1007/978-3-032-29299-5

This Palgrave Macmillan imprint is published by the registered company Springer Nature Switzerland AG
The registered company address is: Gewerbestrasse 11, 6330 Cham, Switzerland

Foreword

Throughout history and throughout the world, minorities and minority communities have been marginalized, ostracized, isolated—and worse. As documented in countless historical studies, Jewish individuals and communities have been particularly vulnerable to various forms of oppression and persecution, repeatedly subjected to prejudices, humiliation, and attacks imposed by dominant societies in which they have lived. Though perhaps less well-documented, disabled individuals and communities, including autistic and other excluded populations, have been consistently victimized by majority groups whose intolerance and insecurities are often manifested through stigmatization and dehumanization of those who are different.

Against this backdrop, evaluating the experience of Jewish individuals on the autism spectrum in contemporary American society is an area of considerable complexity. To be sure, Jewish individuals and communities in the United States have enjoyed a degree of acceptance and belonging virtually unparalleled among thousands of years of Jewish history. Concomitantly, American attitudes toward autism and other disabilities have evolved, incorporating a significant measure of awareness and inclusion that stands as a model for much of the world. Still, biases remain, both explicit and implicit, finding expression in both subtle and more obvious forms of cultural insensitivity and discrimination.

In my work as an advocate for disability rights and inclusion, and through my research on Jewish communities, I have found, anecdotally, that Jewish individuals on the autism spectrum are often placed, along with their families, in a precarious position. Like most others seeking supports and services, Jewish parents of children on the autism spectrum are largely limited to resources available through the public-school system. At the same time, in many geographical areas in the United States, the public-school system adopts Christian religious and cultural norms and assumptions, further marginalizing Jewish students and their families.

Dr. Beth L. Raiola has now presented empirical grounds to help capture the feelings voiced by many Jewish parents and children confronting a lack of ethnic and cultural understanding within public settings. On the basis of research that examines the experience of Jewish families across the United States, Dr. Raiola reaches the conclusion that there is a lack of cultural and social connections within public educational and autism services settings. Moving forward, this study will serve as a powerful resource, motivating ongoing efforts among educators, service providers, administrators, and the broader community, working together to better promote autism awareness, acceptance, and inclusion for all segments of American society.

March 2026

Samuel J. Levine, J.D., LL.M.
Touro Law Center
Long Island, New York, USA

Competing Interests The author has no competing interests to declare that are relevant to the content of this manuscript.

Contents

About the Author

Dr. Beth L. Raiola is a progressive Board-Certified Behavior Analyst licensed in multiple states. Her diverse experience spans schools, clinics, communities, and home settings, working with children and adults with developmental delays, trauma, and neurodiversities. She founded and operated her own agency supporting families with children with autism and other diagnoses, facilitated community partnerships, published articles, delivered talks on child development, taught at several universities, and trained and supported professionals in the field.

Currently, Dr. Raiola serves as Program Chair for Applied Behavior Analysis at Post University and as a contributing faculty member at other institutions. She also provides private training, supervision, mentorship, and workshops for behaviorists and educators working with exceptional learners. Dr. Raiola has served on the Human Services Advisory Committees for Jose Maria Vargas University and Colorado State University. She was also a member of the Nominating Committee for FLAEYC (the Florida Association for the Education of Young Children).

Dr. Raiola is a neurodiversity-affirming, child-centered, and culturally proficient professional dedicated to fostering inclusive environments. She advocates building culturally responsive community partnerships and networks and establishing inclusive systems that foster positive behavioral support, collaborative problem-solving, and individualized opportunities for success.

List of Tables

CHAPTER 1

The Landscape

Abstract Culturally responsive educational and social support programs significantly influence parents' perceptions of support and the quality of service delivery. A relationship has been identified between Jewish American parents' perceptions of culturally responsive education and support, and their consistency with programming for children with autism. Effectively educating and supporting Jewish American children with autism requires a broad perspective and an understanding of cultural diversity for families who share a collective identity. In the United States, the public education system has embodied Christian-based practices and ideologies. Jewish Americans appear to have blended into a White, Christian society and, therefore, as an ethnic and religious minority, maintain a distinct cultural identity that is not always visible or understood.

Keywords Jewish American · Parents · Autism · Culturally responsive · Quality of service · Education

Culturally responsive educational and social support programs significantly influence parents' perceptions of support and the quality-of-service delivery. Research suggests a clear relationship between parental perceptions of culturally responsive education and supports, and their adherence to programming for children with autism (Avery et al., 2022; Gholipour

B. L. Raiola, *Jewish American Parents Navigating Autism Supports*, https://doi.org/10.1007/978-3-032-29299-5_1

et al., 2022). Educating and treating children with autism requires a broad and nuanced understanding of cultural diversity—even among those who share the same racial background. American public education, rooted in Christian-based practices and ideologies that reflect the dominant ethnic culture, has perpetuated minority status for Jewish Americans within the education system (Greenblatt & Koss, 2024). Grayson (2023) described the absorption of Jewish Americans into a White Christian hegemonic social fabric, often perceived as a homogeneous group. While Jewish American parents may appear to mirror the dominant White culture, their beliefs, perspectives, and values can differ significantly, reflecting unique concerns as an ethnic and religious minority (Fulton et al., 2024).

The Autism and Developmental Disabilities Monitoring Network (ADDM) reports a global increase in autism prevalence (Li et al., 2022). The prevalence of autism diagnoses rose from 6.7 (one in 150) per 1000 in 2000 to 23.0 (one in 44) in 2018, with boys diagnosed at four times the rate of girls (Ezeh et al., 2023; Maenner et al., 2023). A major CDC study, which sparked nationwide concern, documented a rise in autism diagnoses among 8-year-old children across multiple states (Maenner et al., 2023). Data from the National Health Information Survey (NHIS), a key resource for health data from the noninstitutionalized US population, confirmed a statistically significant increase in autism prevalence nationwide (Li et al., 2022). Autism spectrum disorder (ASD) diagnoses increased nationally from 2017 to 2020, drawing attention to the need for high-quality, culturally responsive education and treatment services to ensure a positive quality-of-life for the autistic population (Li et al., 2022). ASD prevalence among Asian, Black, and Hispanic children was at least 30% higher in 2020 than in 2018, and among White children with an autism diagnosis was 14.6% higher than in 2018 (Maenner et al., 2023). As the number of diagnoses climbs, more culturally responsive resources may be needed to address diverse quality-of-life criteria (Gholipour et al., 2022).

Surveys and data often categorize people as either people of color or non-Hispanic Whites, without recognizing ethnic subgroups, thereby presenting White statistics as a homogeneous population (Misra et al., 2021). Frey (2023) emphasized the importance of using ethnic subgroups and avoiding simplistic dichotomies of Whites versus non-Whites in cultural and ethnic studies. Jewish Americans are frequently perceived as belonging to a homogeneous White population, which fails to acknowledge the cultural specificity needed in educational and social support for families raising children with autism (Grayson, 2023). The influence of culture within support networks has been linked to perceptions of culturally relevant support and service quality (Bi et al., 2022). Knowledge and competency—including spiritual and religious dimensions—are essential for addressing therapeutic needs effectively (Crabtree et al., 2021). When parents perceive their formal social support systems as providing high-quality, culturally relevant services, they are more engaged in their child's education and treatment. This suggests that clinical service providers and special educators require diversity training to increase parental engagement (Gholipour et al., 2022).

Jewish American parents' cultural and ethnic needs are not integrated into public education and treatment programs for their child with autism in the United States. Scholars have explained the notion of othering, which influences whether Jewish Americans are compelled to hide their ethnic identity in various social contexts (Megerman, 2021). Othering implies feeling outside of the mainstream. Implicit biases are noticed throughout dominant cultural practices in most American social structures, through school or treatment center closings, to acknowledging Christmas, Easter, and other Christian holidays, reinforcing the Jewish experience of otherness (Megerman, 2021). Fulton et al. (2024) indicated the need for clinicians to recognize the unique concerns that may be shaped by Jewish Americans' cultural identity. Religious, spiritual, and ethnic dimensions may impact how an individual with autism self-identifies (Hollins et al., 2023). Ethnic identities may influence medical practices, parenting styles, and cultural views of stigma (Hollins et al., 2023; Likhitweerawong et al., 2022; Misra et al., 2021). Parenting styles and responses may reveal a family's cultural orientation and perceptions about their child's diagnosis, involvement and interaction with support services (Gholipour et al., 2022; Hamama, 2022).

Sociodemographic research indicates a rise in Jewish American communities. Of the 7.5 million Jewish Americans, 92% identify as White (Pew Research Center Report: Jewish Americans in 2020, 2021). Three-quarters of Jewish Americans reported that antisemitism has increased over the past 5 years. In addition to experiencing microaggression, overt practices of exclusion, and microinvalidation, Jewish Americans may be minoritized by dominant group ideologies (Megerman, 2021). Non-White students categorized as racially and ethnically minoritized (REM) are overrepresented in special education. Overrepresentation indicates the prevalence of inequities in elementary education, leading to learning gaps between REM and White students (Malone & Ishmail, 2020). Jewish Americans have been dually categorized as minoritized and White, a blended category unrecognized in the literature (Grayson, 2023).

Special education programs, teacher preparation, and clinician training often lack focus on working with Jewish American populations (Fulton et al., 2024; Greenblatt & Koss, 2024; Jury, 2024). Jewish Americans, though perceived as White, may experience otherness when their unique cultural needs are overlooked (Grayson, 2023; Megerman, 2021). Parents of children with autism require diverse educational supports to stay engaged and provide effective parenting. Recognition of Jewish American cultural identity and needs in raising children with autism is largely absent among practitioners and scholars. Unidentified cultural variables may impact behavioral outcomes and goals. Positive quality-of-life outcomes for children with autism are closely linked to organizations that demonstrate cultural responsiveness and inclusivity (Gholipour et al., 2022). The present qualitative case study may inform practitioners, educators, parents, and communities about the importance of appropriate, relevant supports and systems for Jewish American families raising a child with autism.

A qualitative case study explored Jewish American parents' perceptions of the cultural and ethnic relevance of public education and treatment received by their children with autism across the United States. Sociodemographic classifications often conflate Whites, disregarding distinctions between Christian and non-Christian identities (Grayson, 2023; Misra et al., 2021). Jewish Americans have historically experienced a sense of otherness within White Christian-dominated culture (Megerman, 2021). The literature indicates that parents of children with autism need more intensive support than those of children with other disabilities (Milgramm et al., 2022). Effective parental training should address diverse social and environmental contexts (Schuck et al., 2022). Guidance for parents must reflect child-rearing practices, values, and perceptions, to be truly effective (Danbolt, 2020).

National database researchers substantiated the prevalence of autism has increased significantly over the last decade (Maenner et al., 2023). Quality and culturally responsive social supports are correlated with resilience of parental management and involvement with their developmentally disabled or delayed child, which in turn, impacts the child's externalizing behaviors (Lu et al., 2021). A case study to explore the authentic experiences of Jewish American parents' perceptions of their child's formal social support provided an avenue to enhance service delivery and training of educators, professionals, and caregivers involved in the education and treatment of Jewish American children diagnosed with autism.

Parents of children with autism are involved in numerous networks of support to address a range of challenges common to the autism population, such as co-occurring mental and behavioral health conditions, medical, intellectual, and seizure-related disorders, special education services, speech, occupational, feeding, and physical therapies (Gholipour et al., 2022). Social support networks form a framework that addresses the fundamental needs of parents and impacts their ability to cope, maintain both emotional and physical well-being, and engage (Bi et al., 2022; de la Roche & Im-Bolter, 2024).

Educators and practitioners need more training in working with non-Christian populations in the United States, given Christianity's dominant cultural perspective (Fulton et al., 2024; Greenblatt & Koss, 2024; Jury, 2024). Studies conducted in the United States and United Kingdom highlighted the need for cultural sensitivity, a sense of trust from professionals, and perceived support for parental engagement (Papoudi et al., 2021). Parents raising a child with autism require many social support networks for quality-of-life factors, such as well-being and engagement with their child. Most community programs include training support for parents to develop skills and tools to implement for their child with autism's progress and to improve the quality of their parenting practices (Milgramm et al., 2022; Yan et al., 2022). A strong relationship exists between quality, culturally responsive formal services, and perceived social support, and the well-being of parents raising a child with autism (Bi et al., 2022; Gholipour et al., 2022).

Research on perceptions of culturally relevant support has demonstrated the significance of culture in social support (Gholipour et al., 2022). A qualitative case study provided insight into the needs and experiences of Jewish American parents raising a child with autism (Goh et al., 2021). Implicit biases may contribute to antisemitic practices, which elicit microaggression, evidenced through the dominant cultural practices in most American social structures, which facilitate a Jewish sense of otherness (Megerman, 2021). Active parental involvement in secondary education, explored in Serville, Spain, indicated the essentiality of parental involvement in autism educational support systems for positive academic, social, and developmental outcomes (Fernandez Cecero, 2024). Jewish American parents' perceptions of their children's educators and practitioners engaging in inclusive, culturally relevant support practices may show positive outcomes for their child with autism (Fernández Cerero et al., 2024). Uncovering the needs of Jewish American parents with a child with autism may positively affect change in public educational and equitable treatment practices.

Social support and adaptive leadership ideas shaped this research, which looked at how Jewish American parents feel about the formal service-delivery systems and support they get for their child with autism (Brewer, 2023; Wang et al., 2022). Social support theory highlights the importance of families feeling supported and maintaining a good quality-of-life. Adaptive leadership focuses on making sure leaders create fair, inclusive, and culturally sensitive programs.

There is a link between social support and the conveyance of inclusion, social connectedness, social capital, and well-being (Liamputtong et al., 2022). Social support theory implies the transfer, or perceived transfer, of support from social systems or interpersonal dynamics to satisfy personal needs (Bi et al., 2022). Social capital, or resources, originated in studies on community impact and is equated with social networks (Liamputtong et al., 2022). Formal social support includes public education, medical, psychological, and communal networks. The literature strongly equates a decrease in stress and depression, plus overall improved emotional well-being, with social support received by parents of children with autism (Demšar & Bakracevic, 2023; Yan et al., 2022).

Within social domains, leaders establish policies and protocols. The adaptive leadership approach was based on the notion that people adapt biologically and anthropologically for survival (Heifetz et al., 2009). Contextual challenges of adaptation have been recognized and have stimulated the need to change to assimilate into diverse communities (Glover et al., 2002a). An adaptive leadership orientation evolved from a business perspective and became relevant to public educational and medical institutions, the military, and other milieus (Sunderman et al., 2020).

Adaptive leaders rely on a range of viewpoints and microenvironments and question the status quo (Dunn, 2020; Heifetz et al., 2009). Proponents of adaptive leadership act as integrated members of the group to promote meaningful, systemic change while managing conflict (Dunn, 2020). Informal authority through collaboration is valued, while protecting the change agents to reframe issues and develop adaptive change (Heifetz et al., 2009).

Cultural intelligence is integral to adaptive leadership theory (Azevedo & Jugdev, 2022). A communal mindset projecting one's own cultural viewpoints onto others is a cultural trap (Glover et al., 2002b). Adaptive leadership theory provided a culturally responsive framework to assess Jewish American parents' perceptions of culturally relevant autism supports. Adaptive leadership theory supports a perspective of inclusion and acceptance for implementing and executing programs and for safe exploration through complex transactions (Dunn, 2020). Components recognized for adaptive performance include collaborative systems and unbiased, supportive decision-making (Dunn, 2020).

Adaptive leadership and social support theory guided the exploration of perceptions of Jewish American parents raising a child with autism. The social support lens guided the research on the relationship between autism and high family stress levels and perceptions of holistic, culturally relevant practices across social support systems.

The breadth, extent, or scope of the case study included 13 parents in America who identify as Jewish, raising a child with autism who currently attends or has in the past attended a public elementary school or public middle school in any grade PreK-8 for any part of a school year, and received autism support services. An objective of the study was to ascertain parents' perception of the quality and cultural relevance of public education and formal autism support services.

Snowball sampling was used to recruit parents regardless of region. This determination was made based on the parameters for uncovering a potentially hard-to-reach sample. The outcome of the research may be transferable from dense, rich descriptions, which allow the reader to determine whether the content is relatable to other contexts (Younas et al., 2023). Respondent feedback helped to secure the accuracy of rich, detailed content, contributing to validity, generalizability, and transferability (Terrell, 2023).

The literature provided the building blocks for the open-ended question format, which was developed and implemented. The limitations of conducting a qualitative case study include the data collection method and transferability, as unique participant perceptions were gathered (Henline-Hall, 2024; Lim, 2024; Priya, 2021). Trustworthiness and credibility were solidified from the selection of participants, ensuring their backgrounds aligned with the population. Data were assessed and coded for responses, grouped for relevance and patterns, and bias was continually assessed.

Open-ended questions controlled for potential bias and influence during the interviews (Deroncele-Acosta et al., 2024). Dependability was verified by reviewing interview responses, facilitating debriefing sessions, and member checking for accuracy (Deroncele-Acosta et al., 2024; Lim, 2024). A thorough clarification of the procedure, coupled with a detailed account of the data analysis process, contributed to reliability. The study generated generalizable outcomes for comparable populations across several geographic areas. Further studies may focus on specific regions and demographics. Given the diverse ages and levels of severity of their children, participants in the study had varying years of experience with formal support systems, which did not impact the variability in data outcomes.

National research databases confirm the prevalence of autism has substantially increased over the last decade (Maenner et al., 2023). Survey and interview classifications continue to categorize the White population in America as homogenously Christian (Misra et al., 2021). Hate crimes in Jewish American communities and antisemitism in American public schools (PreK-12) have increased by 100%, and professional training for working with members of the Jewish American community is lacking (Fulton et al., 2024; Hodge & Boddie, 2021). This case study examined Jewish American parents whose child has an autism spectrum disorder and who received formal social support services. The findings arc relevant for community leaders, practitioners, parents, and educators.

Parental involvement in their child's education and treatment may reflect qualitative and culturally relevant formal social supports (Gholipour et al., 2022). Consistent data indicate that children with autism benefit from parental engagement to support progress, positive skill development, and behavioral outcomes (Yan et al., 2022). Quality-of-life measures indicate parental involvement correlates with qualitative social support (Yan et al., 2022). Programs that support and respect family values, traditions, and beliefs are associated with greater family involvement and better outcomes for children with autism (Schuck et al., 2022). There is a strong relationship between raising a child with autism and family quality-of-life, with resources categorized for minority and marginalized cultures and Whites.

Definitions of Terms

Formal social support is defined as funded or governmental, community, or public support such as practitioners, national autism associations, respite services, government-funded and insurance-funded intervention services, state and federally funded educational support or public schools, and other non-denominational services open to the public (Avery et al., 2022; Dunst, 2023).

Informal social support is defined as networks that are not considered official or service organizations but consist of friends, family, or others from within a social network who provide casual assistance (Avery et al., 2022; Dunst, 2023).

Maladaptive cultural traps are defined as the responses within an organizational culture that are considered normalized ways of doing things and are insulated from the external environment (Azevedo & Jugdev, 2022).

Microaggression is defined as communication or behavior that, even if unconscious or unintentional, conveys a prejudiced or biased attitude toward a marginalized person or group (Feaster et al., 2021).

Microinvalidation is a term for communication between a group that reflects an attempt to demean a person's experience, thoughts, or emotions (Parikh & Leschied, 2022).

Minoritized applies to the treatment of those perceived as separate from the dominant group or when a member of a group other than the dominant cultural group is under-represented and lacks recognition (Wingrove-Haugland & McLeod, 2021).

Othering is a term to explain how people who experience being outsiders from the dominant group are treated and their feelings of being separate from the mainstream (Megerman, 2021).

Conflicts of Interest This author has no conflicts of interest to declare that are relevant to the content of this chapter.

References

Avery, K., van Rhijn, T., & Maich, K. (2022). Understanding the role of formal and informal support resources for parent of children with autism spectrum disorder. *Canadian Journal of Family and Youth, 14*(3), 32–51. https://ejournals.library.ualberta.ca/index/php/cify

Azevedo, A., & Jugdev, K. (2022). Applying cultural intelligence to develop adaptive leadership. *Organization Development Journal, 40*(4), 56–70. https://research.ebsco.com/linkprocessor/plink?id=52a7db82-3588-3df3-81badfbc7ce30a90

Bi, X., He, H., Lin, H., & Fan, X. (2022). Influence of social support network and perceived social support on the subjective well-being of mothers of children with autism spectrum disorder. *Frontiers in Psychology, 13*. https://doi.org/10.3389/fpsyg.2022.835110

Brewer, S. (2023). Using adaptive leadership to engage, empower, and energize. *Oncology Practice Management, 13*(1), 1–14. https://research.ebsco.com/linkprocessor/plink?id=50580be1-d871-3355-88f4-5fb470d36f43

Crabtree, S. A., Bell, C. A., Rupert, D. A., Sandage, S. J., Devor, N. G., & Stavros, G. (2021). Humility, differentiation of self, and clinical training in spiritual and religious competence. *Journal of Spirituality In Mental Health, 23*(4), 342–362. https://doi.org/10.1080/19349637.2020.1737627

Danbolt, A. M. V. (2020). Cultural responsiveness in the incredible years parenting program for refugees: A case study. *International Journal of Child Care and Education Policy, 14*(1), 1–19. https://doi.org/10.1186/s40723-020-00071-5

de la Roche, L., & Im-Bolter, N. (2024). A qualitative analysis of parent's perceptions of available social support systems. *Discover Psychology, 4*(1), 1–7. https://doi.org/10.1007/s44202-024-00293-5

Demšar, A., & Bakracevic, K. (2023). Depression, anxiety, stress, and coping mechanisms among parents of children with autism spectrum disorder. *International Journal of Disability, Development and Education, 70*(6), 994–1007. https://doi.org/10.1080/1034912X.2021.1947474

Deroncele-Acosta, A., Gross-Tur, R., Bellido-Valdiviezo, O., & López-Mustelier, R. (2024). Qualitative research from grounded theory to build a scientific framework on the researcher's epistemic competence. *International Journal of Qualitative Methods, 23*, 1–16. https://doi.org/10.1177/16094069241284218

Dunn, R. (2020). Adaptive leadership: Leading through complexity. *International Studies in Educational Administration, 48*(1), 31–38. http://hdl.handle.net/11343/258917

Dunst, C. J. (2023). A meta-analysis of informal and formal family social support studies: Relationships with parent and family psychological health and well-being. *International Journal of Caring Sciences, 16*(2), 514–529. https://doi.org/10.3390/ijerph20186723

Ezeh, T. H., Lee, B. K., & Rast, J. E. (2023). The medical home and use of mental and nonmental specialty services among children with autism spectrum disorder (ASD). *Journal of Autism & Developmental Disorders, 53*(3), 1202–1212. https://doi.org/10.1007/s10803-022-05596-x

Feaster, B., McKinley-Grant, L., & McMichael, A. J. (2021). Microaggressions in medicine. *Cutis, 107*(5), 235–237. https://doi.org/10.12788/cutis.0249
Fernández Cerero, J., Montenegro Rueda, M., & López Meneses, E. (2024). The impact of parental involvement on the educational development of students with autism spectrum disorder. *Children, 11*(9), 1062. https://doi.org/10.3390/children11091062
Frey, T. (2023). Updated guidance on the reporting of race and ethnicity in medical and science journals. *American Medical Writers Association Journal, 38*(1), 36. https://research.ebsco.com/linkprocessor/plink?id=13dae767-0496-31f0-8096-7e95d9888d8c
Fulton, C. L., Melamed, L., & Lambert, A. (2024). Ethno-religious engagement, minority experiences, and strengthening American Jewish identity. *Journal of Mental Health Counseling, 46*(3), 223–258. https://doi.org/10.17744/mehc.46.3.03
Gholipour, K., Ghiasi, A., Shahrokhi, H., Dadashi, Z., Javanmard, S., Tabatabaei, S. H., & Iezadi, S. (2022). Perceptions of the professionals and parents of children with autism spectrum disorders about autism services; a qualitative study. *Journal of Autism and Developmental Disorders, 53*(1), 96–109. https://doi.org/10.1007/s10803-021-05388-9
Glover, J., Friedman, H., & Jones, G. (2002a). Adaptive leadership: When change is not enough (part one). *Organization Development Journal, 20*(2), 15–31. https://www.proquest.com/scholarly-journals/adaptive-leadership-when-change-is-not-enough/docview/198000121/se2
Glover, J., Friedman, H., & Jones, G. (2002b). Adaptive leadership: When change is not enough (part two). *Organization Development Journal, 20*(4), 18–38. https://www.proquest.com/scholarly-journals/adaptive-leadership-part-two-four-principles/docview/197987737/se-2
Goh, J. X., Aishworiya, R., Ho, R. C. M., Wang, W., & He, H. G. (2021). A qualitative study exploring experiences and support needs of parents of children with autism spectrum disorder in Singapore. *Journal of Clinical Nursing, 30*(21–22), 3268–3280. https://doi.org/10.1111/jocn.15836
Grayson, M. L. (2023). Assimilation/appropriation: What Jewish discourses in rhetoric, composition, and writing studies tell us about the limitations of inclusion. *College Composition and Communication, 75*(1), 56–74. https://www.proquest.com/scholarly-journals/assimilation-appropriation-what-jewish-discourses/docview/2897296853/se-2
Greenblatt, D., & Koss, M. D. (2024). Antisemitism as an integral part of anti-bias educational policies and practices. *Journal for Multicultural Education, 18*(4), 385–395. https://doi.org/10.1108/JME-08-2023-0072
Hamama, L. (2022). Perceived social support, normalization, and subjective well-being among family members of a child with autism spectrum disorder.

Journal of Autism and Developmental Disorders. https://doi.org/10.1007/s10803-022-05857-9

Heifetz, R., Grashow, A., & Linsky, M. (2009). *The practice of adaptive leadership: Tools and tactics for changing your organization and the world*. Harvard Business School Publishing. https://doi.org/10.1111/j.1744-6570.2009.01168_4.x

Henline-Hall, J. (2024). Introduction to quantitative and qualitative research methods. *Radiologic Technology, 96*(1), 45–56. https://www.radiologictechnology.org/content/96/1/45.extract

Hodge, D. R., & Boddie, S. C. (2021). Antisemitism in the United States: An overview and strategies to create a more socially just society. *Social Work, 66*(2), 128–138. https://doi.org/10.1093/sw/swab011

Hollins, N. A., Morris, C., & Li, A. (2023). Integrating diversity, equity, and inclusion readings within coursework: Suggestions for instructors teaching behavior analysis. *Behavior Analysis in Practice*. https://doi.org/10.1007/s40617-023-00781-5

Jury, R. T. (2024). Cultural considerations when working with Jewish students and supervisees. *The Clinical Supervisor*, 1–23. https://doi.org/10.1080/07325223.2024.2413060

Li, Q., Li, Y., Liu, B., Chen, Q., Xing, X., Xu, G., & Yang, W. (2022). Prevalence of autism spectrum disorder among children and adolescents in the United States from 2019 to 2020. *JAMA Pediatrics, 176*(9), 943–945. https://doi.org/10.1001/jamapediatrics.2022.1846

Liamputtong, P., Rice, Z. S., & Suwankhong, D. (2022). Social capital and social inclusion. In P. Liamputtong (Ed.), *Handbook of social inclusion* (pp. 43–57). Springer Nature. https://doi.org/10.1007/978-3-030-89594-5_3

Likhitweerawong, N., Boonchooduang, N., & Louthrenoo, O. (2022). Parenting styles, parental stress, and quality of life among caregivers of Thai children with autism. *International Journal of Disability, Development & Education, 69*(6), 2094–2107. https://doi.org/10.1080/1034912X.2020.1837354

Lim, W. M. (2024). What is qualitative research? An overview and guidelines. *Australasian Marketing Journal*, advanced online publication. https://doi.org/10.1177/14413582241264619.

Lu, M., Chen, J., He, W., Pang, F., & Zou, Y. (2021). Association between perceived social support of parents and emotional/behavioral problems in children with ASD: A chain mediation model. *Research in Developmental Disabilities, 113*, 1–9. https://doi.org/10.1016/j.ridd.2021.103933

Maenner, M. J., Warren, Z., Robinson Williams, A., Amoakohene, E., Bakian, A. V., Bilder, D. A., Durkin, M. S., Fitzgerald, R. T., Furnier, S. M., Hughes, M. M., Ladd-Acosta, C. M., McArthur, D., Pas, E. T., Salinas, A., Vehorn, A., Williams, S., Esler, A., Grzybowski, A., Hall-Lande, J., &

Nguyen, R. H. N. (2023). Prevalence and characteristics of autism spectrum disorder among children aged 8 years—Autism and developmental disabilities monitoring network, 11 sites, United States, 2020. *MMWR Surveillance Summaries, 72*(1/2), 1–14. https://doi.org/10.15585/mmwr.ss7202a1
Malone, C. M., & Ishmail, K. Z. (2020). A snapshot of multicultural training in school psychology. *Psychology in the Schools, 57*(7), 1022–1039. https://doi.org/10.1002/pits.22392
Megerman, S. (2021). Voices across the spectrum breaking down "othering" within law librarianship. *American Association of law Libraries (AALL). Spectrum, 26*(2), 38–40. https://research.ebsco.com/linkprocessor/plink?id=0f5d74d6-990b-3193-a3d8-9176340a7aad
Milgramm, A., Corona, L. L., Janicki-Menzie, C., & Christodulu, K. V. (2022). Community-based parent education for caregivers of children newly diagnosed with autism spectrum disorder. *Journal of Autism & Developmental Disorders, 52*(3), 1200–1210. https://doi.org/10.1007/s10803-021-05025-5
Misra, S., Jackson, V. W., Chong, J., Choe, K., Tay, C., Wong, J., & Yang, L. H. (2021). A systematic review of cultural aspects of stigma and mental illness among racial and ethnic minority groups in the United States: Implications for interventions. *American Journal of Community Psychology, 68*(3/4), 486–512. https://doi.org/10.1002/ajcp.12516
Parikh, A. K., & Leschied, J. R. (2022). Microaggressions in our daily workplace encounters: A barrier to achieving diversity and inclusion. *Pediatric Radiology, 52*(9), 1719–1723. https://doi.org/10.1007/s00247-022-05307-9
Pew Research Center. (2021). *Jewish Americans in 2020.* https://www.pewresearch.org/religion/2021/05/11/jewish-americans-in-2020/
Papoudi, D., Jørgensen, C. R., Guldberg, K., & Meadan, H. (2021). Perceptions, experiences, and needs of parents of culturally and linguistically diverse children with autism: A scoping review. *Review Journal of Autism and Developmental Disorders, 8*(2), 195–212. https://doi.org/10.1007/s40489-020-00212-1
Priya, A. (2021). Case study methodology of qualitative research: Key attributes and navigating the conundrums in its application. *Sociological Bulletin, 70*(1), 94–110. https://doi.org/10.1177/0038022920970318
Schuck, R. K., Simpson, L. A., & Golloher, A. N. (2022). How is parental educational involvement related to school satisfaction for parents of young autistic children? *School Community Journal, 32*(1), 201–223. https://research.ebsco.com/linkprocessor/plink?id=69d91d35-d35e-388b-9daeb63424a06803
Sunderman, H. M., Headrick, J., & McCain, K. (2020). Addressing complex issues and crises in higher education with an adaptive leadership framework. *Change, 52*(6), 22–29. https://doi.org/10.1080/00091383.2020.1839322
Terrell, S. R. (2023). *Writing a proposal for your dissertation: Guidelines and examples* (2nd ed.). Guilford Press.

Wang, Z., Wang, L., Chang, S., & Wang, H. (2022). The mediating effect of parenting stress on the relationship between social support and quality of life in parents of children with autistic spectrum disorder: A meta-analytic structural equation modeling. *Frontiers in Psychiatry, 13*, 1–13. https://doi.org/10.3389/fpsyt.2022.713620

Wingrove-Haugland, E., & McLeod, J. (2021). Not "minority" but "minoritized.". *Teaching Ethics, 21*(1), 1–11. https://doi.org/10.5840/tej20221799

Yan, T., Hou, Y., & Deng, M. (2022). The direct, indirect, and buffering effect of social support on parental involvement among Chinese parents of children with autism spectrum disorders. *Journal of Autism and Developmental Disorders, 52*(7), 2911–2923. https://doi.org/10.1007/s10803-021-05170-x

Younas, A., Fàbregues, S., Durante, A., Escalante, E. L., Inayat, S., & Ali, P. (2023). Proposing the "MIRACLE" narrative framework for providing thick description in qualitative research. *International Journal of Qualitative Methods, 22*, 1–13. https://doi.org/10.1177/16094069221147162

CHAPTER 2

The Backstory

Abstract Jewish American parents' perceptions of the cultural and ethnic relevance of public education and treatment for their children with autism in the United States were evaluated. Comprehensive individual and group interviews sought to understand perceptions of formal social supports among Jewish American parents raising and educating a child diagnosed with autism. Notably, there is a lack of research focused specifically on perceptions of culturally responsive supports for Jewish American parents and their children with autism. Research categories do not distinguish variations within White demographic classifications. Published studies have extensively addressed the connection between raising a child with autism and family quality-of-life; research and resources specifically addressing Jewish American families remain limited. Jewish Americans often feel pushed to assimilate into the dominant White culture by playing down their unique identity, disavowing cultural practices, and minimizing visible expressions of their Jewishness. The lack of recognition of Jewish American families' distinct cultures, integral to educative and service delivery practices, may have its roots in microaggression, microinvalidation, and an antisemitic history.

Keywords Cultural and ethnic relevance · Lack of research · Formal social supports · White demographic classifications · Quality-of-life · Distinct culture · Microaggression · Antisemitic

B. L. Raiola, *Jewish American Parents Navigating Autism Supports*,
https://doi.org/10.1007/978-3-032-29299-5_2

An intensive exploration of Jewish American parents' experiences was conducted to ascertain quality-of-life factors and perceptions of social support for raising and educating a child on the autism spectrum. There is a lack of research and information specific to the perception of quality, culturally and ethnically responsive social support received by Jewish American parents for their child with autism. Research categories tend to group ethnic and racial minorities homogeneously, without variation within classifications for Whites (Misra et al., 2021). Published studies have extensively addressed the link between raising a child with autism and family quality-of-life, with resources for minority and marginalized cultures and Whites.

Diversity studies are inclined to separate White from non-White populations, with non-Whites further categorized into subgroups. Jewish Americans are considered an assimilated population; their specific identity is perceived as out of the realm of multiculturalism and, therefore, overlooked (Fulton et al., 2024; Grayson, 2023). The dominant White culture of the American education and health systems maintains a Christian orientation (Grayson, 2023; Greenblatt & Koss, 2024). American public education has embodied Christian-based practices and ideologies, perpetuating minority status for non-Christians (Greenblatt & Koss, 2024; Sher et al., 2022). The problem is that Jewish American parents' cultural and ethnic needs are not integrated into public education and treatment programs for their child with autism.

Research on Jewish Americans' perceptions of social, educational, and community supports and resources to meet their cultural requirements in raising a child with autism is scarce. Sher et al. (2022) reported no previous research on perceptions of stigma of autism in Jewish communities. The prevalence of autism in America has risen in the past decade (Maenner et al., 2023). Prevalence estimates of 8-year-olds with an autism diagnosis per 1000 children was 27.6, an increase from prior estimates from the ADDM Network (Maenner et al., 2023). Statistical categories were broken down for Blacks and Hispanics, with all non-Hispanics categorized as Whites (Maenner et al., 2023). As formal autism diagnoses continue to rise, more culturally responsive support resources are needed to meet the diverse quality-of-life criteria (Gholipour et al., 2022).

Leaders with adaptive leadership orientations can foster inclusivity and culturally relevant practices within public education and formal social support systems (Brewer, 2023). Adaptive leadership theory and social support theory are relevant for exploring systems of support pervading the lives of parents raising a child with autism. Parents raising children with autism tend to be members of multicomponent support networks (Bi et al., 2022). Social support theory was applied to explore American Jewish parents' perceptions of social support for raising a child with autism.

Proponents of a social support perspective have reported a correlation between raising a child on the autism spectrum and high family stress levels. Social support theory evolved from the development of a network system of social control and criminality (Cullen et al., 1999). Multiple dimensions of social support include perceived support (feeling supported), instrumental support (tangible assistance), and sources of support such as family, systems, schools, religious institutions, community, and other secondary groups (Bi et al., 2022). Applying the social support perspective highlights the central role of the family, the capacity to cope with stress, and the promotion of psychological and physical well-being (Bi et al., 2022; Dunst, 2023). Research on social support theories has shown a correlation between positive social support and quality-of-life (Hamama, 2022). Both emotional and physical parental stress levels have been linked to the perceived quality of social support (Bi et al., 2022; Yan et al., 2022). Psychological stress may be exhibited by parents who perceive the service delivery from social support structures as inadequate (Hamama, 2022; Wang et al., 2022). Positively perceived social support networks and resources were associated with more positive attitudes and interactions between parents and their children with autism (Yan et al., 2022).

Leaders who implement adaptive strategies promote equitable active collaboration by recognizing psychological, social, cultural, and contextual barriers to change (Hogan, 2008). Adaptive leaders recognize core beliefs and cultural traps that affect decision-making and behavior (Hogan, 2008). Within healthcare and education, leaders continue to evaluate, and develop policies for equity, diversity, and inclusion (Kuluski et al., 2021; Sunderman et al., 2020). The professional development of leaders in education and healthcare highlighted the need for additional training and coursework working with Jewish populations (Fulton et al., 2024). The adaptive leadership process, viewed as sociological, recognizes culture traps, knowledge management, synergy, and inclusive, holistic practices across social support systems (Azevedo & Jugdev, 2022; Jefferies, 2017). Leaders who adopt the adaptive approach join their teams to help them adapt to changes and embrace new realities

(Brewer, 2023). Adaptive leaders assess the larger picture to understand root causes while applying a deep understanding of cultural components (Brewer, 2023).

Contextual challenges of adaptation have been recognized, prompting the need to adapt to diverse communities (Glover et al., 2002a). Assimilation as a concept originated with the foundational work of Piaget and was subsequently applied to organizational contexts (Glover et al., 2002a). The ability to meld and grow to survive within their environment becomes successful through accommodation and assimilation (Glover et al., 2002a). Adaptive leadership helps guide people through change and encourages real, positive improvements in society (Glover et al., 2002a).

Cultural intelligence is integral to adaptive leadership (Azevedo & Jugdev, 2022). With cultural traps in mind, the capacity for accommodation without assimilation arises when the leader makes a profound change without the full scope of critical information, resulting in ineffectiveness (Glover et al., 2002b). Leaders can discern patterns from a broader perspective, identify gaps in values, attitudes, beliefs, and behaviors, and create a holding environment that facilitates adaptive work (Heifetz et al., 2009). Reformed thinking and behavior are adopted to address contextual demands through assimilation and accommodation, while relying on diverse viewpoints (Azevedo & Jugdev, 2022; Heifetz et al., 2009).

Adaptive leaders recognize when people rely on traditional ways of doing things and are open to trying new approaches to see what is most effective (Heifetz et al., 2009). Leaders challenge the status quo and, while stepping back, integrate as group members to facilitate substantial, systemic change while controlling conflict (Dunn, 2020). Collaboration is fostered through informal authority that protects the voices of change agents, enabling them to reframe issues and develop not simply technical change but adaptive change (Heifetz et al., 2009).

Inequities are assessed, core beliefs are examined, and norms shift to change behaviors and relationships as adaptive leaders rise (Kuluski et al., 2021). Culturally responsive social support to meet the needs of parents for their child with autism within the hidden, diverse Jewish culture requires the willingness of social structures to be reframed from ideologies rooted in Christianity. Adaptive leaders maintain a mindset of inclusivity and acceptance to drive action, program development, and safe risk-taking in evolving, complex situations (Dunn, 2020).

There is a relationship between social support and the human transmission of culture, material, and social capital at the interpersonal and macro levels (Cullen et al., 1999). Social support theory grew from studies of criminality and antisocial behavior, focusing on the quality of social connections (Cullen et al., 1999). Central to social support theory is the delivery or perceived delivery of help from social systems or interpersonal relationships to meet personal needs (Bi et al., 2022). The elements impacting the health and well-being of individuals include the interrelatedness of social connectedness or a sense of belonging, social capital or access and quality of resources, and social inclusion or the ability to participate and cultivate relationships (Liamputtong et al., 2022).

Social support is defined as tangible, instrumental, informational, and emotional, and is measured by received and perceived social support (Bi et al., 2022). Elements that comprise social support are positively correlated with social, psychological, and physical health (Bi et al., 2022). Studies on social support and overall well-being have provided substantial evidence that social support and social ties are linked to improved physical and mental health.

Types of social structures within social support networks include the formal service category and informal support (Avery et al., 2022; Dunst, 2023). Social ties comprise informal systems such as family, friends, and neighbors. Formal supports are described as professional and structured organizations. Formal social support includes educational, medical, psychological, and communal (Dunst, 2023). Parents of children with autism experience significant decreases in stress and depression, along with increased parental engagement and adaptive coping, when they receive social support (Demšar & Bakracevic, 2023).

Parents are expected to be involved in treatment through caregiver collaboration sessions and learn behavior skill strategies to improve their child's symptoms (Rohacek et al., 2023). There is consistency in the research on the positive outcomes of parental involvement in the education and treatment of youngsters with autism (Yan et al., 2022). There is a strong correlation between qualitative and culturally responsive formal services and perceived social support and well-being of mothers of children with autism (Bi et al., 2022; Gholipour et al., 2022). Research on the function of culture within social support networks has demonstrated the significance of perceptions of qualitative, culturally relevant supports (Avery et al., 2022; Gholipour et al., 2022). Overall, family quality-of-life is impacted by the external and autism support services received (Wang et al., 2022).

Jewish American parents' perceptions of their formal social support for their child with autism were engaged to share whether their needs within a culturally responsive context were met. Within social support systems, decision-makers influence policies, programs, and practices. In formal social support systems, adaptive leadership practices need to be assessed in relation to Jewish American parents' perceptions of culturally relevant service delivery for their child with autism.

Jewish American parents with a child with autism may have a distinct culture and ethnicity, potentially affecting educators, therapists, and practitioners' adaptive ability to meet the needs of this undistinguished minority (Flasch & Fulton, 2019). Quality-of-life issues and perceptions of social support for parents raising and educating a child with autism were examined. There is a gap in the literature specific to the perception of quality, culturally and ethnically relevant social support received by Jewish American parents for their child with autism.

Jewish American parents, classified as White, may have a distinct culture and ethnicity, which has been overlooked by the medical and educational community, potentially making Jewish parents an invisible minority (Flasch & Fulton, 2019). The purpose of analyzing the literature was to explore whether Jewish American parents perceived that the public education and treatment received for their child, with autism, met their needs culturally and ethnically.

There is a greater proclivity of stress in parents raising a child with autism than in other developmental disabilities (Sneed & Samelson, 2022). Parents experienced high levels of stress and were confronted with enormous challenges in finding high-quality autism services (Gholipour et al., 2022). Qualitative formal social support, including educational, medical, and therapeutic, tended to decrease the negative impact of the demands of raising a child with autism (de la Roche & Im-Bolter, 2024). Studies on resiliency confirmed that when parents perceived lack of social support for their child with neurodevelopmental disabilities, their resilience for managing and interacting with their child was diminished, which influenced the child's externalizing behaviors (Lu et al., 2021). Parents of children with autism have felt anxious, depressed, hopeless, low levels of well-being, and minimal parenting self-efficacy (de la Roche & Im-Bolter, 2024; Milgramm et al., 2022). Social support services for parents and their children with autism are vital (Lu et al., 2021; Yan et al., 2022).

Criteria for assigning an autism diagnosis have widened to include previously categorized diagnoses, such as Asperger syndrome, childhood disintegrative disorder, and pervasive developmental disorder—not otherwise specified (PDD-NOS) (American Psychiatric Association, 2022). Symptoms among those with autism have been assigned severity specifiers from one to three, requiring little (one) to most (three) levels of support (American Psychiatric Association, 2022). Parents' ability to handle stress depends on multiple factors (Bi et al., 2022). Children on the autism spectrum may present challenges such as social and behavioral deficits, communication limitations, and inflexibility in thought and behavior (Wang et al., 2022). Parents with children with ASD need support due to stress contributions to depression, anxiety, and emotional fatigue, likely impacting family interactions (Demšar & Bakracevic, 2023).

Ongoing parental participation in their child's education and treatment for autism is essential for developmental outcomes (Sneed & Samelson, 2022; Yan et al., 2022). Parental involvement in their child's programs is correlated with the relationships and quality of support parents feel from the professionals and their informal support systems (Avery et al., 2022; Wang et al., 2022). Perceptions of their child's care impact emotional well-being, influencing parents' ability to cope and provide positive parenting. Formal and informal social supports were associated with parents' motivation and acceptance of their child's diagnosis (Avery et al., 2022). Family quality-of-life has been determined congruent with the availability of qualitative resources, emotional, financial, educational, and social supports. (Gholipour et al., 2022; Schuck et al., 2022). Interventions and supports are vital to relieving the stress and emotional strain of parenting a child with a developmental disability and assisting parents with adaptive coping skills (Sneed & Samelson, 2022; Yan et al., 2022).

Children with more severe levels of autism require more intensive services, including occupational therapy, speech therapy, physical therapy, feeding therapy, and, at all severity levels, are typically receiving applied behavior analytic services (Dallman et al., 2021). More severe symptomatology was associated with a greater likelihood of co-occurring diagnoses, exacerbating deficits (Dallman et al., 2021). Children in the United States diagnosed with autism are regularly identified as having an assortment of unmet healthcare needs than children with other developmental diagnoses (Dallman et al., 2021). Parents fulfill multiple roles for their child with autism as caregivers, advocates, and educators, with high parental involvement and demand an integral aspect of their daily lives (Avery et al.,

2022). There is a recognized need for strong family support through informal social support systems to combat intense levels of stress and anxiety experienced in raising a child with autism and to enhance coping skills (Yan et al., 2022).

The importance of parental involvement at the onset of the diagnostic process is indisputable (Gholipour et al., 2022). Parents of a child with autism, a lifelong condition, may require multiple dimensions of support to appraise their individual experiences as supportive and culturally responsive (Hamama, 2022; Sher et al., 2022). Service providers who communicated sensitively and engaged parents in their child's treatment were perceived as providing high-quality, effective support (Gholipour et al., 2022; Yan et al., 2022). Professional interventions with parental engagement have been shown to contribute to positive outcomes for children with autism (Gholipour et al., 2022). Challenges faced by children with autism range in severity, profoundly impacting a family's overall well-being. Solid formal (and informal) social networks enhanced a sense of parental competence or self-efficacy in addressing challenges and reduced pressure and negative impacts (Lu et al., 2021; Sneed & Samelson, 2022). Family quality-of-life stressors are not confined to the parents but may also affect siblings, circuitously compounding parental psychosocial factors of emotional health, including anxiety and depression (Hamama, 2022).

Strong social networks were linked to parenting confidence (Lu et al., 2021). Mothers who perceived their social support networks as positive conveyed subjective well-being (Bi et al., 2022). Quality social support reduces stress by acting as a buffer, moderating the relationship between parental stress and involvement. Parental stress and child autism outcomes confirm the need for parental engagement, which can be demanding and time-intensive (Sneed & Samelson, 2022; Yan et al., 2022). Research confirms a strong connection between effective social support and improved emotional well-being, positive quality-of-life factors, greater parental efficacy, and stronger parent-child relationships. These factors are critical for the developmental progress of children with autism (Yan et al., 2022).

Ethnic minority parents experienced challenges with cultural factors during the diagnostic process (Gholipour et al., 2022). Parents reported a lack of culturally competent application of diagnostic tools, judgmental biases, and cultural differences between professionals and Iranian parents (Gholipour et al., 2022). Structural and organizational challenges and poor management added to parents' ability to perceive qualitative care for their child with autism (Gholipour et al., 2022).

Caregivers in South Africa reported experiencing discrimination and social isolation and avoided social events due to stigmatization and embarrassment. Caregivers claimed there was a lack of social awareness, knowledge, and comprehension surrounding autism and the accompanying parental struggles (Dira et al., 2024). The stigma of autism in communities in the United Kingdom was uncovered (Sher et al., 2022). It has been claimed that cultural perspectives influence stigma and autism (Dira et al., 2024). In Jewish communities in the United Kingdom, some parents refrained from taking their child with autism to synagogue and expressed strong fears of stigmatization (Dira et al., 2024). Commonalities among cultural studies included social stigmatization, cultural barriers, challenges in working with professionals and diagnosticians, and a lack of knowledge among parents and communities about autism (Papoudi et al., 2021). A lack of information about autism and discerning stigmatization influence caregivers' perceptions of quality support systems, impacting parental self-efficacy, involvement, and engagement (Sneed & Samelson, 2022).

Parent training and education are vital to involvement with the child's programs. When parents of a child with autism felt supported, feelings of isolation lessened, and parents were able to broaden their pool of resources (Hamama, 2022). It has been suggested that the level of support needed for parents of a child on the autism spectrum is more intense than for those with other disabilities (De la Roche & Im-Bolter, 2024). Parent coaching and implementation of parent interventions are critical for positive outcomes and must be taught using diverse social and environmental contexts (Sneed & Samelson, 2022). Creating culturally relevant parental programs and using implementation research to inform feedback on parental application is necessary (Dawson-Squibb & de Vries, 2019).

Cultural adaptation models of diverse populations were used to monitor parents' needs to reduce cultural barriers to implementation. Guidance for parents may take many shapes, but must include factors related to upbringing practices, values, and perceptions to be effective (Danbolt, 2020). Cultural and linguistic considerations were examined in a parenting program aimed at integrating a multicultural refugee population into Norwegian society; culture was defined as a conglomerate of behaviors, artifacts, norms, values, everyday activities, and experiences (Danbolt, 2020). Parental involvement in medical and educational programs has been repeatedly assessed for cultural relevance as a critical component, particularly for parents with a child with autism (Fernández Cerero et al., 2024; Gholipour et al., 2022).

Linking parents to social support services for their children with autism is essential for promoting emotional well-being and improving family quality-of-life (Dunst, 2023). Parental involvement and acceptance are especially important, as parents raising a child with a developmental disability often face significant stressors (Sher et al., 2022). Chassidic mothers raising children with autism experienced feelings of isolation and emphasized the importance of both community and parental social support. (Levy & Mulcahey, 2017). The literature highlights that Jews are often depicted as an invisible minority, with comparative research on the ethnic identity process of Jewish Americans in a predominantly Christian society revealing a persistent sense of otherness (Fulton et al., 2024).

The size of Jewish communities in the United States has grown over the past several decades (Pew Research Center, 2021). Most Jewish Americans define their identity primarily through ancestry or culture rather than religious observance (Fulton et al., 2024). There are approximately 7.5 million Jewish Americans, with 92% identifying as White (Pew Research Center, 2021). Notably, three-quarters of Jewish Americans have reported an increase in antisemitism over the past five years.

In examining the behaviors and practices of contemporary Jewish Americans, it was discovered that although many do not actively participate in religious institutions, they often experience a strong emotional connection to both local and global Jewish communities, as well as to Israel (Fulton et al., 2024). Jewish American identity is complex and multifaceted, with most individuals declaring more connectedness to Jewish culture than to religious practices. The Pew Research Center (2021) study found that while Jewish Americans express pride in their heritage, a relatively small percentage are engaged in Judaic community life, though strong cultural and historical ties remain prevalent.

Across denominational affiliations—Orthodox, Conservative, Reform, or Secular—Jewish Americans share a sense of common Jewish identity (Fulton et al., 2024). This identification is often reinforced through time spent with family and Jewish friends, as well as participation in Jewish social circles (Bankier-Karp, 2023). Engaging in Jewish holidays, rituals, life-cycle events, traditional meals, and learning about Jewish history and origins fortifies Jewish identity irrespective of level of religiosity or observance (Fulton et al., 2024). Many Jewish Americans are unaffiliated with formal Jewish institutions, which may explain why their strong Jewish connection may be overlooked (Fulton et al., 2024). Jewish Americans express a strong cultural identity, shaped by shared minority experiences and antisemitic events. Informal social support networks, particularly through family ties, are common among Jewish American parents, potentially contributing to less engagement with formal social support systems (Abrams & Wertheimer, 2021). Despite varying degrees of secularity, Jewish Americans commonly identify with a shared ancestry, culture, and a collective history of persecution, leading to a profound sense of solidarity in response to antisemitism (Hodge & Boddie, 2021).

Cultural Bias in Formal Support Services

American Jewish communities experienced a rise of approximately 54% in hate crimes between 2014 and 2017, and antisemitism in American public schools (K-12) increased by 100%, according to a 2018 study by the Anti-Defamation League (Hodge & Boddie, 2021). Christian ideologies are embedded in public education programs, reinforce minority status for non-Christians, and permeate psychosocial support programs (Dupper et al., 2015). Teachers' attitudes toward inclusion and inclusive practices, known as the teacher factor, influence the type of students who experience inclusion. It was found that non-Christian students experience macroaggressions, reinforced by prevailing Christian practices in the school, which lead to feelings of non-inclusivity (Dupper et al., 2015). The prevailing American belief system rests on Protestant Christian religious ideology, which impacts religious inclusion among public school leaders (Pfaff et al., 2021). Conservative Protestantism, as the overarching lens, has deemed valid American values as synonymous with American nationalism, with intolerance for minorities or atheists (Pfaff et al., 2021).

A smaller number than the dominant population indicates minority-group status (Wingrove-Haugland & McLeod, 2021). Members of a group other than the dominant cultural group as under-represented do not address effects, hence the term minoritized (Wingrove-Haugland & McLeod, 2021). In addition to experiencing microaggression, overt practices of exclusion, and microinvalidation, Jewish Americans may be minoritized by dominant group ideologies (Pfaff et al., 2021). Othering, feeling outside the mainstream, has influenced whether Jewish Americans hide their ethnic identity in various social contexts (Megerman, 2021). Implicit biases are evident in the dominant cultural practices within most American social structures that acknowledge seasonal holidays such as Christmas and Easter, reinforcing the Jewish sense of otherness (Megerman, 2021).

The significance and ethics of ethnic and cultural awareness have been recognized in the counseling professions (Fulton et al., 2024). There is a lack of scholarship and training among clinicians to address specific Jewish considerations shaped by their distinct spiritual and cultural backgrounds (Fulton et al., 2024). Researchers acknowledged an increase in racial, ethnic, and culturally minoritized populations, with a projected rise to 50% of children under 18 in the United States by the year 2060 (Malone & Ishmail, 2020). Inequities in elementary education have led to learning gaps between White students and those categorized as racially and ethnically minoritized (REM) who are overrepresented in special education (Malone & Ishmail, 2020).

Jewish Americans have been categorized as both minoritized and White, a combined and unrecognized category (Malone & Ishmail, 2020). Cultural competency in school psychologists' training remains essential for developing proficiency in working with multiple cultural identities and for developing awareness of implicit biases (Malone & Ishmail, 2020). Behavior analysts are professionals who are typically part of the interdisciplinary treatment or education team of children with autism. Behavior analysts provide applied behavior analysis methods in their work with learners with autism, and the demand for this service delivery has accelerated due to the success for children with autism and their parents (Hollins et al., 2023). Hollins et al. (2023) recommended that training and graduate programs in applied behavior analysis include diversity, equity, and inclusion courses, with a primary focus on marginalized populations.

Variables indicating the relationship between demographics and outcomes of behavioral goals may be needed for culturally responsive modifications in treatment and education for the child with autism (Jones et al., 2020). Cultural variables not identified in research might impact behavioral outcomes and goals (Jones et al., 2020). The notion of cultural competency in helping professions, including spiritual and religious competency, is suggested (Crabtree et al., 2021). Knowledge and skills for competency extend beyond culture to include spiritual and religious dimensions, thereby positively addressing therapeutic needs. Education and training on clinical protocols require integrating spiritual and religious diversity, which may impact behavioral engagement (Crabtree et al., 2021). Research in applied behavior analysis has historically lacked diversity and demographic reporting (Hollins et al., 2023). Ethical and culturally responsible practices require ethical self-knowledge through self-reflection. Behaviorally therapeutic orientations require culturally responsive practices for conducting assessments, developing behavior plans, and integrating cultural variables into humanistic programs (Hollins et al., 2023). Cultural, spiritual, ethnic, and religious dimensions impact on how individuals with autism self-identify and how parents respond to their child's diagnosis (Hollins et al., 2023).

Parenting styles and responses reflect a family's cultural orientation and can influence perceptions about their child's diagnosis, involvement, and interaction with services (Hamama, 2022; Likhitweerawong et al., 2022). A meaningful pathway for positive quality-of-life measures that foster a parent's ability to advocate for, interact with, and adhere to critical developmental and behavioral programming for their child's progress is congruent with organizations that exhibit cultural responsiveness and inclusive practices.

Justice, diversity, and inclusion programs, seeking to protect certain minorities, have omitted the Jewish population (Abrams & Wertheimer, 2021). Antisemitism may have its roots in the historical discriminatory practices that Jewish immigrants experienced by White supremacists. In the 1950s, American universities enforced implicit quotas for the enrollment of Jewish students. Contemporary Jewish American leaders and academicians object to being categorized or connected with the White privileged class, claiming their historical and cultural distinctiveness is not recognized (Abrams & Wertheimer, 2021). The concept of microaggression and microinvalidation has been expanded to include minoritizing, which refers to practices that place accountability on the dominant group (Wingrove-Haugland & McLeod, 2021). Prevalent microinvalidations have been expanded to include the experience by Jewish Americans to assimilate into the dominant White culture and hide their unique identity by disavowing practices and erasing their Jewishness (Atadgy, 2022). The effects of direct and indirect bias in patient care have been reported to affect treatment and can lead to internalized damage (Turner et al., 2021).

Positive health outcomes and satisfaction with autism services have been measured by parents' perceptions of their child's culturally responsive care (Jafarabadi et al., 2021). Parenting styles often reflect cultural values and beliefs (Likhitweerawong et al., 2022). Social structures related to education, health, and public institutions require adaptive leadership to assess the root causes of discriminatory, minoritized, and otherness practices that affect the quality of culturally responsive formal social support delivery (Likhitweerawong et al., 2022). Social support theory addresses the value of formal support systems relevant to family quality-of-life and well-being. Effective quality health care is viewed as a public health issue (Jafarabadi et al., 2021). Adaptive leadership embraces the skill set of leaders who evaluate cultural traps, lead with cultural competence, and leverage unconscious biases to adjust social structures and implement new, relevant, and culturally appropriate accommodations (Azevedo & Jugdev, 2022). Leaders of adaptive theory apply a framework to detect the root cause and engage members of an organization to collaborate and interact to uncover and reconfigure processes. Cultural intelligence is a relevant dimension of adaptive leadership theory applicable to unearthing implicit bias at the systemic level within formal social structures.

Counterargument

Raising a child with developmental disabilities, particularly autism, has impacted physical and psychological stress, well-being, and quality-of-life (de la Roche & Im-Bolter, 2024; Demšar & Bakracevic, 2023). Parents of a child with autism from all cultural backgrounds may experience similar emotional challenges. Social support may be perceived as qualitative or inadequate, irrespective of cultural background with little difference between American Jewish parents' perceptions of services from other parents with a child with autism.

A recent Pew Research Center (2021) study reported Jewish Americans either identified as Orthodox and enmeshed in a religious community or the opposite, with no practice or religious affiliation. Twenty-seven percent of Jewish Americans do not identify with the religion (Pew Research Center Report: Jewish Americans in 2020,, 2021). As a result, American Jewish parents who have assimilated into the dominant White culture may not perceive themselves as having particular or unique needs unmet by their formal social supports. Jewish Americans have been perceived as maintaining stable family lives and investing in their children

(Abrams & Wertheimer, 2021). The Jewish American family is regarded as the anchor, generating confident members of American society. It may be that Jewish Americans' informal social support continues to provide a strong family quality-of-life despite the stressors of raising a child with autism.

Whether overt or implicit, interpersonal, or social discrimination correlates with health and well-being, people of color in America who fall outside of a White racial group identity, including Blacks, Latinos, Indigenous, Asian Americans, native Hawaiians, and Pacific Islanders, may face consistent discrimination and cultural unresponsiveness across service-delivery systems (Serchen et al., 2021). Assimilation and adaptation to the dominant White culture may have enabled Jewish Americans to integrate with fewer challenges and experience less obvious minoritization (Atadgy, 2022). Consequently, formal social service systems in education and healthcare for Jewish parents of a child with autism may be less culturally unresponsive, with fewer disparities than those for people of color.

The literature reviewed the significance of qualitative social support services, and resources for parents with a child with autism. Scholars and researchers indicated a correlation between raising a child with autism and psychological and physical wellness and quality-of-life (Sneed & Samelson, 2022). Little has been found in the literature targeting Jewish American parents' needs, raising a child with autism, distinct from the dominant culture based on White Christian ideologies (Dupper et al., 2015). Adaptive leadership and social support orientations provided a lens to explore links between parental perceptions of Jewish American parents with a child with autism and qualitative social support to meet their needs through culturally responsively led service systems (Panopoulos & Drossinou-Korea, 2020).

Community, educational, and therapeutic systems of support are essential for parents with a child with autism to ensure active involvement in their child's developmental, behavioral, and emotional needs (Hayes et al., 2023; Yan et al., 2022). Research suggested that parents who remained involved in their child's education and treatment saw significant developmental progress (Yan et al., 2022). Programs must appeal to parents' cultural and ethnic affiliations to help them feel understood and supported by formal service-delivery organizations (Gholipour et al., 2022; Papoudi et al., 2021).

A qualitative case study provided information for professionals, parents, and communities on the need for building appropriate, relevant supports, resources, and social systems for Jewish American parents raising a child with autism. Jewish American parents may require systemic change to ensure supports align with their unique values, culture, and practices. Research does not differentiate data among White populations, potentially failing to identify the distinct culturally specific needs of Jewish American families (Misra et al., 2021).

This author has no conflicts of interest to declare that are relevant to the content of this chapter.

References

Abrams, S. J., & Wertheimer, J. (2021). The woke threat to America—And to American Jews. *Commentary, 152*, 17. https://research.ebsco.com/linkprocessor/plink?id=70e14f5b-e68b-3138-b8e0-71d60d873089

American Psychiatric Association. (2022). *Diagnostic and statistical manual of mental disorders* (5th ed., text rev.). https://doi.org/10.1176/appi.books.9780890425787

Atadgy, R. Z. (2022). Denying Jewish identity is the epitome of anti-semitism: Radical politics is forcing a false and wicked choice on American Jews. *Commentary, 153*(6), 34–38. https://research.ebsco.com/linkprocessor/plink?id=0d30e707-056d-380c-94de-16a40a7d49cc

Avery, K., van Rhijn, T., & Maich, K. (2022). Understanding the role of formal and informal support resources for parent of children with autism spectrum disorder. *Canadian Journal of Family and Youth, 14*(3), 32–51. https://ejournals.library.ualberta.ca/index/php/cify

Azevedo, A., & Jugdev, K. (2022). Applying cultural intelligence to develop adaptive leadership. *Organization Development Journal, 40*(4), 56–70. https://research.ebsco.com/linkprocessor/plink?id=52a7db82-3588-3df3-81badfbc7ce30a90

Bankier-Karp, A. L. (2023). Catalysts of connectedness: Three wellsprings of Jewish culture and their effects on Jewish cultural identity. *Review of Religious Research, 65*(2), 165–192. https://doi.org/10.1177/0034673X231187779

Bi, X., He, H., Lin, H., & Fan, X. (2022). Influence of social support network and perceived social support on the subjective well-being of mothers of children with autism spectrum disorder. *Frontiers in Psychology, 13*, 835110. https://doi.org/10.3389/fpsyg.2022.835110

Brewer, S. (2023). Using adaptive leadership to engage, empower, and energize. *Oncology Practice Management, 13*(1), 1–14. https://research.ebsco.com/linkprocessor/plink?id=50580be1-d871-3355-88f4-5fb470d36f43

Crabtree, S. A., Bell, C. A., Rupert, D. A., Sandage, S. J., Devor, N. G., & Stavros, G. (2021). Humility, differentiation of self, and clinical training in spiritual and religious competence. *Journal of Spirituality In Mental Health, 23*(4), 342–362. https://doi.org/10.1080/19349637.2020.1737627

Cullen, F. T., Wright, J. P., & Chamlin, M. B. (1999). Social support and social reform: A progressive crime control agenda. *Crime & Delinquency, 45*(2), 188–207. https://doi.org/10.1177/0011128799045002002

Dallman, A. R., Artis, J., Watson, L., & Wright, S. (2021). Systematic review of disparities and differences in the access and use of allied health services amongst children with autism spectrum disorders. *Journal of Autism & Developmental Disorders, 51*(4), 1316–1330. https://doi.org/10.1007/s10803-020-04608-y

Danbolt, A. M. V. (2020). Cultural responsiveness in the incredible years parenting program for refugees: A case study. *International Journal of Child Care and Education Policy, 14*(1), 1–19. https://doi.org/10.1186/s40723-020-00071-5

Dawson-Squibb, J. J., & de Vries, P. J. (2019). Developing an evaluation framework for parent education and training in autism spectrum disorder: Results of a multi-stakeholder process. *Journal of Autism & Developmental Disorders, 49*(11), 4468–4481. https://doi.org/10.1007/s10803-019-04176-w

de la Roche, L., & Im-Bolter, N. (2024). A qualitative analysis of parent's perceptions of available social support systems. *Discover Psychology, 4*(1), 1–7. https://doi.org/10.1007/s44202-024-00293-5

Demšar, A., & Bakracevic, K. (2023). Depression, anxiety, stress, and coping mechanisms among parents of children with autism spectrum disorder. *International Journal of Disability, Development and Education, 70*(6), 994–1007. https://doi.org/10.1080/1034912X.2021.1947474

Dira, P. M. M., Machailo, R. J., & Scholtz, S. (2024). Caregivers' voices: From the world of autism spectrum disorder. *Curationis, 47*(1), 1–11. https://doi.org/10.4102/curationis.v47i1.2519

Dunn, R. (2020). Adaptive leadership: Leading through complexity. *International Studies in Educational Administration, 48*(1), 31–38. http://hdl.handle.net/11343/258917

Dunst, C. J. (2023). A meta-analysis of informal and formal family social support studies: Relationships with parent and family psychological health and well-being. International Journal of Caring Sciences, 16(2), 514–529. https://doi.org: 10.3390/ijerph20186723.

Dupper, D. R., Forrest-Bank, S., & Lowry-Carusillo, A. (2015). Experiences of religious minorities in a public-school setting: Findings from focus groups involving Muslim, Jewish, Catholic, and Unitarian universalist youths. *Children & Schools, 37*(1), 37–45. https://doi.org/10.1093/cs/cdu029

Fernández Cerero, J., Montenegro Rueda, M., & López Meneses, E. (2024). The impact of parental involvement on the educational development of students with autism spectrum disorder. *Children, 11*(9), 1062. https://doi.org/10.3390/children11091062

Flasch, P., & Fulton, C. L. (2019). Counseling Jewish Americans: Considerations for practice. *Counseling and Values, 64*, 2–19. https://doi.org/10.1002/cvj.12091

Fulton, C. L., Melamed, L., & Lambert, A. (2024). Ethno-religious engagement, minority experiences, and strengthening American Jewish identity. *Journal of Mental Health Counseling, 46*(3), 223–258. https://doi.org/10.17744/mehc.46.3.03

Gholipour, K., Ghiasi, A., Shahrokhi, H., Dadashi, Z., Javanmard, S., Tabatabaei, S. H., & Iezadi, S. (2022). Perceptions of the professionals and parents of children with autism spectrum disorders about autism services; a qualitative study. *Journal of Autism and Developmental Disorders, 53*(1), 96–109. https://doi.org/10.1007/s10803-021-05388-9

Glover, J., Friedman, H., & Jones, G. (2002a). Adaptive leadership: When change is not enough (part one). *Organization Development Journal, 20*(2), 15–31. https://www.proquest.com/scholarly-journals/adaptive-leadership-when-change-is-not-enough/docview/198000121/se2

Glover, J., Friedman, H., & Jones, G. (2002b). Adaptive leadership: When change is not enough (part two). *Organization Development Journal, 20*(4), 18–38. https://www.proquest.com/scholarly-journals/adaptive-leadership-part-two-four-principles/docview/197987737/se-2

Grayson, M. L. (2023). Assimilation/appropriation: What Jewish discourses in rhetoric, composition, and writing studies tell us about the limitations of inclusion. *College Composition and Communication, 75*(1), 56–74. https://www.proquest.com/scholarly-journals/assimilation-appropriation-what-jewish-discourses/docview/2897296853/se-2

Greenblatt, D., & Koss, M. D. (2024). Antisemitism as an integral part of anti-bias educational policies and practices. *Journal for Multicultural Education, 18*(4), 385–395. https://doi.org/10.1108/JME-08-2023-0072

Hamama, L. (2022). Perceived social support, normalization, and subjective well-being among family members of a child with autism spectrum disorder. *Journal of Autism and Developmental Disorders, 54*(4), 1468–1481. https://doi.org/10.1007/s10803-022-05857-9

Hayes, K. N., Rossetti, K. G., & Zlomke, K. (2023). Community support, family resilience and mental health among caregivers of youth with autism spectrum disorder. *Child: Care, Health & Development, 49*(1), 130–136. https://doi.org/10.1111/cch.13025

Heifetz, R., Grashow, A., & Linsky, M. (2009). *The practice of adaptive leadership: Tools and tactics for changing your organization and the world*. Harvard Business School Publishing. https://doi.org/10.1111/j.1744-6570.2009.01168_4.x

Hodge, D. R., & Boddie, S. C. (2021). Antisemitism in the United States: An overview and strategies to create a more socially just society. *Social Work, 66*(2), 128–138. https://doi.org/10.1093/sw/swab011

Hogan, T. J. (2008). The adaptive leadership maturity model. *Organization Development Journal, 26*(1), 55–61. https://www.proquest.com/scholarly-journals/adaptive-leadership-when-change-is-not-enough/docview/198000121/se-2?accountid=31683

Hollins, N. A., Morris, C., & Li, A. (2023). Integrating diversity, equity, and inclusion readings within coursework: Suggestions for instructors teaching behavior analysis. *Behavior Analysis in Practice, 16*(2), 629–639. https://doi.org/10.1007/s40617-023-00781-5

Jafarabadi, M. A., Gholipour, K., Shahrokhi, H., Malek, A., Ghiasi, A., Pourasghari, H., & Iezadi, S. (2021). Disparities in the quality of and access to services in children with autism spectrum disorders: A structural equation modeling. *Archives of Public Health, 79*(1), 1–11. https://doi.org/10.1186/s13690-021-00577-5

Jefferies, S. S. (2017). Adaptive leadership in a socially revolving world: A symbolic interactionist lens of adaptive leadership theory. *Performance Improvement, 56*(9), 46–50.

Jones, S. H., St Peter, C. C., & Ruckle, M. M. (2020). Reporting of demographic variables in the *journal of applied behavior analysis*. *Journal of Applied Behavior Analysis, 53*(3), 1304–1315. https://doi.org/10.1002/jaba.722

Kuluski, K., Reid, R. J., & Baker, G. R. (2021). Applying the principles of adaptive leadership to person-centered care for people with complex care needs. *Health Expectations, 24*(2), 175–181. https://doi.org/10.1111/hex.13174

Levy, F., & Mulcahey, M. J. (2017). Examining the experiences and unmet needs of Chassidic mothers raising a child with autism. *American Journal of Occupational Therapy, 17*, 1–3. https://doi.org/10.5014/ajot.2017.71S1-PO4058

Liamputtong, P., Rice, Z. S., & Suwankhong, D. (2022). Social capital and social inclusion. In P. Liamputtong (Ed.), *Handbook of social inclusion* (pp. 43–57). Springer Nature. https://doi.org/10.1007/978-3-030-89594-5_3

Likhitweerawong, N., Boonchooduang, N., & Louthrenoo, O. (2022). Parenting styles, parental stress, and quality of life among caregivers of Thai children with autism. *International Journal of Disability, Development & Education, 69*(6), 2094–2107. https://doi.org/10.1080/1034912X.2020.1837354

Lu, M., Chen, J., He, W., Pang, F., & Zou, Y. (2021). Association between perceived social support of parents and emotional/behavioral problems in children with ASD: A chain mediation model. *Research in Developmental Disabilities, 113*, 1–9. https://doi.org/10.1016/j.ridd.2021.103933

Maenner, M. J., Warren, Z., Robinson Williams, A., Amoakohene, E., Bakian, A. V., Bilder, D. A., Durkin, M. S., Fitzgerald, R. T., Furnier, S. M., Hughes, M. M., Ladd-Acosta, C. M., McArthur, D., Pas, E. T., Salinas, A., Vehorn, A., Williams, S., Esler, A., Grzybowski, A., Hall-Lande, J., & Nguyen, R. H. N. (2023). Prevalence and characteristics of autism spectrum disorder among children aged 8 years—Autism and developmental disabilities monitoring network, 11 sites, United States, 2020. *MMWR Surveillance Summaries, 72*(1/2), 1–14. https://doi.org/10.15585/mmwr.ss7202a1

Malone, C. M., & Ishmail, K. Z. (2020). A snapshot of multicultural training in school psychology. *Psychology in the Schools, 57*(7), 1022–1039. https://doi.org/10.1002/pits.22392

Megerman, S. (2021). Voices across the spectrum breaking down "othering" within law librarianship. *American Association of Law Libraries (AALL) Spectrum, 26*(2), 38–40. https://research.ebsco.com/linkprocessor/plink?id=0f5d74d6-990b-3193-a3d8-9176340a7aad

Milgramm, A., Corona, L. L., Janicki-Menzie, C., & Christodulu, K. V. (2022). Community-based parent education for caregivers of children newly diagnosed with autism spectrum disorder. *Journal of Autism & Developmental Disorders, 52*(3), 1200–1210. https://doi.org/10.1007/s10803-021-05025-5

Misra, S., Jackson, V. W., Chong, J., Choe, K., Tay, C., Wong, J., & Yang, L. H. (2021). A systematic review of cultural aspects of stigma and mental illness among racial and ethnic minority groups in the United States: Implications for interventions. *American Journal of Community Psychology, 68*(3/4), 486–512. https://doi.org/10.1002/ajcp.12516

Panopoulos, N., & Drossinou-Korea, M. (2020). Bronfenbrenner's theory and teaching intervention: The case of a student with intellectual disability. *Journal of Language and Linguistic Studies, 16*(2), 537–551. https://doi.org/10.17263/jlls.759243

Papoudi, D., Jørgensen, C. R., Guldberg, K., & Meadan, H. (2021). Perceptions, experiences, and needs of parents of culturally and linguistically diverse children with autism: A scoping review. *Review Journal of Autism and Developmental Disorders, 8*(2), 195–212. https://doi.org/10.1007/s40489-020-00212-1

Pew Research Center. (2021). *Jewish Americans in 2020.* https://www.pewresearch.org/religion/2021/05/11/jewish-americans-in-2020/

Pfaff, S., Crabtree, C., Kern, H. L., & Holbein, J. B. (2021). Do street-level bureaucrats discriminate based on religion? A large-scale correspondence experiment among American public school principals. *Public Administration Review, 81*(2), 244–259. https://doi.org/10.1111/puar.13235

Rohacek, A., Baxter, E. L., Sullivan, W. E., Roane, H. S., & Antshel, K. M. (2023). A preliminary evaluation of a brief behavioral parent training for challenging behavior in autism spectrum disorder. *Journal of Autism & Developmental Disorders, 53*(8), 2964–2974. https://doi.org/10.1007/s10803-022-05493-3

Schuck, R. K., Simpson, L. A., & Golloher, A. N. (2022). How is parental educational involvement related to school satisfaction for parents of young autistic children? *School Community Journal, 32*(1), 201–223. https://research.ebsco.com/linkprocessor/plink?id=69d91d35-d35e-388b-9daeb63424a06803

Serchen, J., Doherty, R., Atiq, O., & Hilden, D. (2021). A comprehensive policy framework to understand and address disparities and discrimination in health and health care: A policy paper, *American college of physicians. Annals of Internal Medicine, 174*(4), 529–532. https://doi.org/10.7326/M20-7219

Sher, D. A., Gibson, J. L., & Sher, H. E. (2022). "We've come a very, very, long way" overcoming stigma of autism: An interpretative phenomenological analysis within the UK Jewish community. *Autism: The International Journal of Research & Practice, 26*(8), 2066–2083. https://doi.org/10.1177/13623613221075099

Sneed, L., & Samelson, D. (2022). Effectiveness of parent-led applied behavior analysis at improving outcomes for parents of autistic children. *Journal of Social, Behavioral & Health Sciences, 16*(1), 160–177. https://doi.org/10.5590/JSBHS.2022.16.1.12

Sunderman, H. M., Headrick, J., & McCain, K. (2020). Addressing complex issues and crises in higher education with an adaptive leadership framework. *Change, 52*(6), 22–29. https://doi.org/10.1080/00091383.2020.1839322

Turner, J., Higgins, R., & Childs, E. (2021). Microaggression and implicit bias. *The American Surgeon, 87*(11), 1727–1731. https://doi.org/10.1177/00031348211023418

Wang, Z., Wang, L., Chang, S., & Wang, H. (2022). The mediating effect of parenting stress on the relationship between social support and quality of life in parents of children with autistic spectrum disorder: A meta-analytic structural equation modeling. *Frontiers in Psychiatry, 13*, 1–13. https://doi.org/10.3389/fpsyt.2022.713620

Wingrove-Haugland, E., & McLeod, J. (2021). Not "minority" but "minoritized.". *Teaching Ethics, 21*(1), 1–11. https://doi.org/10.5840/tej20221799

Yan, T., Hou, Y., & Deng, M. (2022). The direct, indirect, and buffering effect of social support on parental involvement among Chinese parents of children with autism spectrum disorders. *Journal of Autism and Developmental Disorders, 52*(7), 2911–2923. https://doi.org/10.1007/s10803-021-05170-x

CHAPTER 3

Lived Experiences: A Case Study

Abstract There is a clear need to develop appropriate and relevant supports that guide Jewish American parents toward meaningful resources aimed at improving their quality-of-life and that of their children with autism. Employing case study methodology facilitated the collection of rich information through narrative inquiry, useful for exploring parental perceptions of autism support service systems among Jewish American parents whose child with a diagnosis of autism attends or has attended a public elementary or middle school (PreK–8) and has received autism support services. In-depth individual and group interviews encapsulated parents' perceptions of whether formal services met their children's needs and were culturally relevant.

Keywords Relevant supports · Meaningful resources · Case study · Interviews · Formal services · Culturally relevant

The dominant White culture of the American education and health systems maintains a Christian orientation (Dupper et al., 2015). There is a potential need for building appropriate, relevant supports to guide Jewish American parents toward access to meaningful resources to improve their quality-of-life and that of their child with autism. Case study practices align to support the collection of information about people, phenomena,

B. L. Raiola, *Jewish American Parents Navigating Autism Supports*,
https://doi.org/10.1007/978-3-032-29299-5_3

and social processes (Prosek & Gibson, 2021). A case study remains relevant for analyzing and synthesizing perspectives on a particular issue in real-life contexts (Rogo, 2024). Narrative inquiry of social phenomena was useful for studying parental perceptions of autism support service systems (Lim, 2024).

Case studies that use an interview process foster understanding of human experiences and can be more collaborative and inclusive among facilitators and participants (Akingbola & Brunt, 2023). The case study interview process can elicit details about participants' cultures and foster cultural responsiveness and collaboration (Naeem et al., 2023; Prosek & Gibson, 2021). A case study was conducted with the intent to inform practitioners, educators, parents, and communities on the potential need for building appropriate, relevant supports, resources, and social systems for Jewish American parents with a child with autism. This endeavor was a valid approach for social inquiry and to provide storied data to discover and make connections among perceptions and experiences (Priya, 2021; Younas et al., 2023).

The population consisted of Jewish American parents whose child with autism who attends or has in the past attended a public elementary or middle school in any grade, PreK-8, for any part of a school year, and received autism support services.

In-depth interviews captured parents' perceptions of whether formal services were meeting their children's needs and were culturally relevant. An open interview process was conducted in an atmosphere of acceptance to make sense of how Jewish American parents raising children with autism perceive their social challenges through lived experiences (Lim, 2024).

Semi-structured and unstructured interview questions and a focus group were extended to invite Jewish American parents with a child with autism, involved in public education and service-delivery support systems, to share their perceptions. Participants were asked to sign informed consent declarations that clarified the purpose, research design and process, inclusion criteria, the voluntariness of participation, and the option to withdraw or refuse participation. Interviews and focus group discussions unfolded collaboratively, creating an environment of reciprocity, engagement, involvement, and trust (Akingbola & Brunt, 2023).

Outcomes from the case study on the perceptions of Jewish American parents raising a child with autism can provide justification for the need to build appropriate, relevant systems to guide access to meaningful resources. The case study approach provides an effective method of inquiry for examining complex issues in social phenomena and human experiences (Lim, 2024). This was applicable for studying parental perceptions of autism support service systems through an exploratory inquiry into social phenomena in a relevant real-world context (Lim, 2024). Case study interviews examine social change and complex human and social phenomena and acknowledge individuals' voices and perspectives through a human-centered approach (Lim, 2024). The study was built around clear problems and a purpose, and it set out specific questions to guide the research. Interviews and focus groups were carefully planned to ensure the process was ethical and trustworthy.

This case study can help teachers, professionals, and communities understand the needs of Jewish American parents to better support their children with autism. Case studies are useful for looking at real-life situations and hearing different perspectives. The study included interviews with 13 Jewish American parents whose children with autism received support services and currently attend or previously attended public school. Parents were asked open-ended questions about whether these services met their child's needs while respecting their culture.

Methodology and Research Procedures

The study used open and respectful interviews to understand parents' views. Instead of focusing on numbers and data, this approach is about hearing people's stories and learning how they see the challenges they face.

Qualitative research was chosen because it helps us understand people's experiences and allows participants to share their lived experiences. Other methods, such as ethnographic or grounded theory, didn't fit this study's goals because they require more time or focus on developing new theories rather than gathering parents' feedback on culturally responsive autism supports.

Parents were invited to share their experiences through interviews and a focus group. They received information about the study and were free to decide whether to participate. The interviews and group discussions fostered open and honest sharing, providing valuable insights into families' experiences with autism services and supports.

The case study focused on hearing directly from parents about how well autism support and schooling meet their cultural needs. Interviews were conducted in a conversational, friendly manner to ensure parents felt comfortable sharing their genuine opinions. The study kept all parts—questions, methods, and analysis—focused on this main goal. The study used a clear process, starting with picking participants through referrals, then interviewing and running focus groups, and finally analyzing the results. Every step was taken carefully and respectfully, in accordance with ethical guidelines.

Population and Sample Selection

The population consisted of Jewish American parents whose child with autism attends or has in the past attended a public elementary or middle school in any grade, PreK-8, for any part of a school year, and received autism support services.

The first 13 respondents who met the criteria comprised the sample; a small sample size is adequate for data collection, providing rich and extensive descriptions (Rogo, 2024; Younas et al., 2023). The sample size supported one-on-one and focus group interviews, through transcriptions from the virtual Zoom platform and member checking (Terrell, 2023).

Snowball sampling is purposeful for identifying participants and useful for involving participants in recruiting others (Terrell, 2023). A bounded system, or a system targeting a particular group to gain understanding within their frame of reference, yielded data that informed the findings and contributed to snowball sampling. Potential participants were contacted to clarify the steps in the research process. Each potential participant was invited to refer parents who met the inclusive screening criteria and might be interested in contributing to the study. The snowball sampling process continued until data collection reached saturation (Terrell, 2023).

Follow-up outreach included full disclosure and clarification of the study's purpose and the instrumentation. A request was provided to the participants to review and sign an informed consent to participate and allow for video recording via DocuSign or hand-signed and returned by email. A one-to-one Zoom time was set up. Participants were asked if they would be interested in participating in a 20–30 minute focus group following the interview.

A friendly and safe environment was provided using motivational interviewing skills including open-ended questions, affirmation, compassion, and active, reflective listening (Miller & Rollnick, 2023). The need for privacy and the lack of distractions during the virtual interviews were explained to ensure a safe and confidential environment. The identities of the one-on-one interview participants were kept anonymous using pseudonyms instead of name identifiers. Focus group participants' identities were not disclosed in any documentation.

Data Collection

Data collection occurred through an online Zoom platform of researcher-generated interview questions and focus group topics. Interviewees were requested to participate from a quiet, private location. A review of informed consent and privacy protocols was reiterated prior to administering a systematic approach (Capili & Anastasi, 2024). Orienting questions provided the opening or introduction, using a motivational interviewing style to convey interest in the interviewees' perspectives through active listening, compassion, and affirmation, establishing a collaborative dynamic and laying the groundwork (Miller & Rollnick, 2023). Unstructured questions were used as prompts to elicit elaborate descriptive responses aligned with the research questions. Roberts (2020) referred to these main questions as the "grand tour," as they encourage the participants to piece together their experiences with effusive details.

Follow-up questions ensued using active and reflective listening strategies as issues and aspects of the responses emerged (Miller & Rollnick, 2023; Roberts, 2020). Interviewing is a fluid, flexible process, and in uncovering individual perceptions of the population's lived experiences, probing questions develop through the researcher's active listening (Miller & Rollnick, 2023). Self-reflective and reflexive behaviors emerged, using affirmative body language and responses such as nodding or verbalizations, "Please continue." Participants' responses and reflexivity indicated when to dig deeper, probe further, or when expanded details were warranted (Akingbola & Brunt, 2023). After each interview, a succinct debrief with the interviewee ensued to collaborate. Participants of the focus group maintained a conversational dialogue with guided topics. The focus groups were conducted on Zoom, with permission to record. Transcription data from online recordings contributed to robust data collection.

Data Preparation

Interviews conducted in a one-on-one format and focus group discussions contributed to the data. The data were transcribed in the setup or open coding phase, labeled using pseudonyms, which were employed throughout analyses, and organized into encrypted, password-protected electronic files. Once transcribed from the Zoom cloud recorded transcripts, the data were coded to construct meaning and relevance in an organized fashion (Rogo, 2024). A progressive coding process ensured that the responses correlated with the interview questions. All data from interviews and focus groups were read for familiarization, comparison, and recognition of themes from the textual data (Braun & Clarke, 2022). The process, known as open coding, yielded theme fragments sorted into broad categories based on repeated words, phrases, and content from the responses (Lim, 2024;Lochmiller, 2021; Naeem et al., 2023).

Compiling all collected data enabled the first phase of preparing and organizing all responses (Naeem et al., 2023). Continuously reviewing the transcribed data generated a familiarity with the individual and group narratives, developing patterns and themes. The data were checked for accuracy using member checking or respondent feedback to ensure that participants' authentic responses were appropriately captured (Terrell, 2023). All responses were prepared by sorting codes that represented trends and patterns (Naeem et al., 2023). The answers provided by the participants that reflected meaning and constructed rich case significance provided thematic integration as the process unfolded. Codes were assigned to respondents' perceptions as patterns, and shared stories emerged throughout phases of data analysis (Lochmiller, 2021; Naeem et al., 2023).

All interview and focus group transcripts were reviewed for familiarity, comparison, and theme recognition, and sorted into broad categories by identifying recurring words, phrases, and content from the responses (Braun & Clarke, 2022; Naeem et al., 2023). Compiling the collected narratives facilitated the preparation and organization of responses (Naeem et al., 2023). Five emerging themes and subthemes were uncovered from the one-on-one interviews (see Table 3.1).

Thematic display from the individual interviews.

Overall themes emerged from the focus groups that supported those uncovered from the one-on-one interviews. Three prevailing themes emerged within the focus groups (see Table 3.2).

Table 3.1 Prominent themes and subthemes from one-on-one interviews

Themes	*Subthemes*	*Participant quotes*
Public education	Quality of education	*"His academics are way above grade level, so they don't care. There's just not enough support for inclusion."*
Autism services	Quality of services	*"They're very open. If there's something I don't like or something I don't think we need to work on yet. They're very open to my suggestions."*
Parent advocacy	Advocate for educational and cultural relevance	*"I was actually a very involved parent. And so, like, I helped to start that inclusion program in the public school."*
Jewish supports	Jewish identity, and community	*"We follow the religion fully. In normal circumstances our kids would have all gone to religious Jewish schools. It wasn't appropriate for him, which is why he wasn't there. But that's how we live."*
Christian-dominant culture	Awareness of diversity from school and services	*"He hears a lot of Christmas normativity, brings home art projects, and I asked them not to do that, but it still happens. The calendar revolves around Christian holidays...bombarded with Christmas."*

Table 3.2 Prominent themes and subthemes from focus group interviews

Themes	*Subthemes*	*Participant quotes*
Public education	Responsiveness to autism diagnosis; getting an IEP	*"...it took me until 7th–8th grade to get an IEP."*
Christian-dominant culture	Jewish parents' cultural awareness attempts	*"they're* [her children] *pretty familiar with the holidays and traditions...so they want to bring those things to school, like I ask the teachers every year, do you mind if I send some dreidels? I have a write up that I offer to send, if the teachers wanted to explain the holiday."*
Jewish supports	Jewish identity and Jewish community	*"My son will tell you that this is the place where he feels the most accepted, for who he is, and always knows that he belongs."*

Thematic display generated from individual interviews.

An extensive examination revealed patterns across respondents' thematic fragments and perceptions (Lochmiller, 2021; Naeem et al., 2023). Evolving thematic analytic models offered a trustworthy and profound approach to assigning meaning to lived experiences derived from the case study (Saunders et al., 2023; Terrell, 2023).

Parents stressed the need to adapt to ensure optimal services and educational opportunities for their children. Instead of expecting service providers or educators to possess in-depth cultural awareness, parents primarily sought acceptance and respect—achieved through their own advocacy. Above all, addressing their children's needs was paramount, transcending considerations of religiosity or ethnicity. Parents reported that their cultural needs were generally fulfilled outside of public education or service systems.

Conflicts of Interest This author has no conflicts of interest to declare that are relevant to the content of this chapter.

References

Akingbola, K., & Brunt, C. (2023). Reflexivity in nonprofit management research: A reflection on the role of self as researcher. *Nonprofit Management & Leadership, 34*(2), 465–479. https://doi.org/10.1002/nml.21564

Braun, V., & Clarke, V. (2022). *Thematic analysis: A practical guide*. Sage.

Capili, B., & Anastasi, J. K. (2024). Ethical research and the institutional review board: An introduction. *American Journal of Nursing, 124*(3), 50–54. https://doi.org/10.1097/01.NAJ.0001008420.28033.e8

Dupper, D. R., Forrest-Bank, S, & Lowry-Carusillo, A. (2015). Experiences of religious minorities in a public-school setting: Findings from focus groups involving Muslim, Jewish, Catholic, and Unitarian universalist youths. *Children & Schools, 37*(1), 37–45. https://doi.org/10.1093/cs/cdu029

Lim, W. M. (2024). What is qualitative research? An overview and guidelines. *Australasian Marketing Journal*, advanced online publication. https://doi.org/10.1177/14413582241264619

Lochmiller, C. R. (2021). Conducting thematic analysis with qualitative data. *The Qualitative Report, 26*(6), 2029–2044. https://doi.org/10.46743/2160-3715/2021.5008

Miller, W. R., & Rollnick, S. (2023). *Motivational interviewing helps people change* (4th ed.). Guilford Press.

Naeem, M., Ozuem, W., Howell, K., & Ranfagni, S. (2023). A step-by-step process of thematic analysis to develop a conceptual model in qualitative research. *International Journal of Qualitative Methods, 23*, 1–18. https://doi.org/10.1177/16094069231205789

Priya, A. (2021). Case study methodology of qualitative research: Key attributes and navigating the conundrums in its application. *Sociological Bulletin, 70*(1), 94–110. https://doi.org/10.1177/0038022920970318

Prosek, E. A., & Gibson, D. M. (2021). Promoting rigorous research by examining lived experiences: A review of four qualitative traditions. *Journal of Counseling & Development, 99*(2), 167–177. https://doi.org/10.1002/jcad.12364

Roberts, R. E. (2020). Qualitative interview questions: Guidance for novice researchers. *The Qualitative Report, 25*(9), 3185–3203. https://doi.org/10.46743/2160-3715/2020.4640

Rogo, E. J. (2024). Exploring qualitative research. *Journal of Dental Hygiene, 98*(4), 56–61. https://api.semanticscholar.org/CorpusID:271862404

Saunders, C. H., et al. (2023). Practical thematic analysis: A guide for multidisciplinary health services research teams engaging in qualitative analysis. *BMJ, 381*, 1–10. https://doi.org/10.1136/bmj-2022-074256

Terrell, S. R. (2023). *Writing a proposal for your dissertation: Guidelines and examples* (2nd ed.). Guilford Press.

Younas, A., Fàbregues, S., Durante, A., Escalante, E. L., Inayat, S., & Ali, P. (2023). Proposing the "MIRACLE" narrative framework for providing thick description in qualitative research. *International Journal of Qualitative Methods, 22*, 1–13. https://doi.org/10.1177/16094069221147162

CHAPTER 4

Shared Narratives

Abstract Analysis of all interview and focus group narratives revealed distinct patterns and themes. Recurring words, phrases, and topics emerged among parents' responses, and a comprehensive review of these stories unveiled shared experiences. Themes and subthemes were identified from both one-on-one interviews and focus groups, as parents openly discussed their lived experiences with public education and service delivery. Consistent themes included fostering their child's Jewish identity within a societal context dominated by a White Christian social fabric, limited opportunities for social skills development and socialization, a strong commitment to advocacy, and the recognition that their child's autism-related needs and services often took precedence over other aspects of their ethnic, cultural, or religious life, regardless of the parents' level of Jewish observance.

Keywords Distinct patterns · Consistent themes · Jewish identity · Limited opportunities for social skills · Commitment to advocacy · Autism-related needs

The educational and treatment support serving autism populations in the United States has assumed a standard that aligns with a White Christian cultural fabric. There is a gap in published research addressing Jewish

B. L. Raiola, *Jewish American Parents Navigating Autism Supports*,
https://doi.org/10.1007/978-3-032-29299-5_4

American parents' perceptions of the cultural relevance and quality of their child's public education and autism support services. The cultural and ethnic needs of Jewish American parents are overlooked in public education and treatment programs for children with autism. To explore this issue, Jewish American parents of children with autism were interviewed to understand their perceptions regarding whether educational and social support services met their expectations for quality and cultural responsiveness. Their rich stories yielded shared narratives and common themes derived from experiences as Jewish American parents of children with autism receiving support services and public schooling.

One-on-One Interviews

Theme 1. Public Education

Parents indicated that their child on the autism spectrum encountered difficulties in the school setting during the early years. Most of their children had delays or behavioral challenges that caused concerns. Some had an older child on the spectrum, so they knew the signs. Others identified deficits, but educators and physicians did not initially attribute the issues to a specific diagnosis. Two participating families received an autism diagnosis for their child at 3 and 4 years of age. Most parents struggled to receive an IEP for their child, and the average age of diagnosis of autism for the participants' children was age six. Parents expressed the need to advocate for their children's educational programs and were actively involved in educating, advising, and guiding school administrators and educators on their children's needs. Children who did not exhibit cognitive or intellectual disabilities ran "under the radar" despite having social, emotional, or behavioral deficits. Parents needed to convince schools to provide evaluations, IEPs, or to locate a psychologist for further assessments, even to ascertain an autism diagnosis. They championed their children and secured accurate and appropriate academic placement.

Theme 2. Autism Services

Children of the participants currently receive, or have received throughout their school years, support services such as speech, behavioral therapy, occupational and/or physical therapy, counseling, and social skill groups. Parents found autism services relevant and helpful at various stages of their child's development. Many of their children's continued goals contained a social skills component. Parents spoke favorably about their autism services; those received at the school were less impactful, such as speech, occupational, and behavior therapy, which, when obtained privately, was more individualized and qualitative.

Social skills groups were consistently identified by parents interviewed as a primary need for the children. Schools, usually through speech programs, provide social skills groups.

"...we could see that he was struggling socially with sustaining and maintaining friendships...and he would say he was lonely and couldn't just didn't understand." Parents conveyed a lack of opportunities for social interactions and felt that a meaningful community, such as after-school clubs or parent events, was lacking. One parent expressed dissatisfaction with the school's social skills group, which she felt did not meet her child's needs. Social skills were best supported in programs outside the school setting with a Jewish component. Parents consistently reported a sense of acceptance in Sunday school programs and culturally related programs, independent of school.

Theme 3. Parent Advocacy

Participating parents were active crusaders for their children with autism. Committed advocacy for their children was attributed to a Judaic upbringing and Jewish values. In communities where Jewish connections were minimal, parents either found small communities or started Jewish support groups for families with children with autism. Schools were sought that accommodated their child's needs. Most of the children attended multiple schools until their parents found the best fit for their child's special education and autism support needs. Parents did not accept the school's or service provider's lack of responsiveness when IEPs were needed, or the diagnosis was ignored. Most observant parents, who identified as Orthodox or Modern Orthodox and typically sent their children to Yeshiva, put their observant practices on "the back burner." Children from observant families attended a public school that provided more resources and more rigorous, targeted autism education and support.

Theme 4. Jewish Supports

The families represented various denominations of Judaism: Orthodox, Modern Orthodox, Conservative, Reform, and Secular. Parents consistently expressed the "we certainly grew up with a very Jewishly connected plan," although that was adapted differently depending upon the families' level of observance. Consensus among participating parents, however, was a belief in "separation of church and state" and that "it's not their responsibility to teach my child his religious and cultural heritage. That's my responsibility." Parents educated the schools by supplying ethnic treats for Jewish holidays or requesting that winter programs include Hanukkah when speaking of Christmas. One Orthodox mother stated,

"We follow the religion fully. In normal circumstances, our kids would have all gone to religious Jewish schools. It wasn't appropriate for him, which is why he wasn't there. But that's what we're about." Regarding public school, "it was very much an atmosphere of inclusivity; there was no judgment. And it really was such a positive experience. Our biggest issue, I would say one of the big ones, is kosher food." When there were birthday parties, for kosher accommodations, "either a teacher will go out and buy something specifically for him, or at least they will let us know in advance, so that we can provide something." Her son's affiliation with his Jewish identity ensured her that, even in a public-school setting, he would know if the food was not kosher, not to eat it.

All but one family indicated that their child felt connected to their Jewish identity; however, all are preparing, intend to prepare, or have given their child a Bar/Bat Mitzvah. Parents who did not live in a community with any or a small number of other Jewish families opted to start their own support groups. One participant and local Jewish parents of a child with autism started a Bar/Bat Mitzvah preparation program after speaking with various rabbis, and it became so popular that it evolved into a non-profit organization. Since there is a lack of Jewish programs for children like his son, a participant decided to attempt to start one in his area.

A parent reported that their children outwardly expressed a rejection of Christmas and Santa in the public-school setting and received negative input from peers and non-teaching staff, and felt that, following the Israeli dissonance of October 7, 2024, her child felt a stronger connection to her Jewish identity. Another parent remarked that, following October 7, 2024, she felt "like being a little more invisible," although she requested

Hanukkah be added to the winter program, she did not pursue it. The commonality among the families, regardless of level of observance, was the importance of being part of a Jewish community and had "gotten most of my support from outside the school setting" as expected. "...outside of school, there were a lot of Jewish assistance with autism that I became involved with...really, all of our autism support has been through Jewish programs."

Parents sought Jewish connections through Jewish organizations such as the JCC and their local synagogues. Three parents felt it was too challenging to engage their children in temple services due to their social skill deficits and behavioral challenges; however, they did provide a level of Jewish education in the home through observance of certain holidays and festivities, lighting candles on the Sabbath, and/or introducing culturally specific holiday foods and books. There was a strong Judaic connection for each family, whether they identified as practicing or Secular, and they wished to provide a Jewish community for their children. Parents found a sense of belonging and support among other Jewish families with a child with autism. "...we have enough people around us who can understand. Enough that we can speak to them.... So we're very lucky to have each other to have those relationships because it makes it easier. On Sunday mornings, I take them for Sunday school. I would just say, I like to chat with friends, and we hang out with coffee.... it's a natural space and place."

Theme 5. Christian Dominant Culture

All participants felt connected to their Jewish culture and ethnicity and attempted to incorporate these values into their children's lives. As public-school parents of a Jewish background, they were cognizant of the lack of programming that incorporated their culture. Two parents have children who attend a public-school that does not normalize one culture, has a diverse, though minimally Jewish, population, and does not acknowledge any celebrations. One of the two parents stated, "I think it's very culturally responsive." None of the parents felt that the Christian-dominant culture, by way of winter shows focusing on Christmas and Christmas music, Christmas crafts, the notion of Santa, and a school calendar that "revolves around Christian holidays" had a negative impact on their child's education or autism support services, which was a strong priority. One parent indicated the cultural aspect wasn't even on their radar as the educational needs were paramount, and the culture was their "last concern." An Orthodox parent shared a heartfelt story about her minimally verbal son who participated in a holiday program that was exclusively centered around Christmas. He was given an opportunity to sing the verse in the Twelve Days of Christmas song, "Five Golden Rings," and, in front of an audience of people, in a sweet and clear voice, sang the words. For this parent of a son with autism, it was a turning-point moment that brought her to tears. The parents conveyed that autism needs and supports were their highest priority. The same parent reported that the school did a great job with her child, who eventually had his Bar Mitzvah, and that all the school personnel and students who supported him, albeit non-Jewish, attended and cheered him on.

Focus Groups

Theme 1. Public Education

Respondents collaborated on their experiences obtaining IEPs for their children with autism. Parents expressed feeling angry when IEPs were delayed. "…we're outraged when a child doesn't have an IEP by age five…to us, it is like, how dare you?" Children were identified as having delays at a young age, and the parents advocated for early intervention services. Many championed for years for an autism diagnosis and a full battery of assessments. One parent pushed their son's school to hire an outside clinical psychologist to finally provide an IEP.

Another participant was a clinician who contacted colleagues in the fields of education and psychology for assistance. Without these connections, she could not ascertain an IEP for her son. She attributed the issue to the district's budget and felt "…they really don't care about special education needs in this city; and I'm not the only parent who has had to fight for IEPs"

Parents in her district had to fight for services such as speech and OT, however, having colleagues in the same field eventually provided an advantage, and her son, with autism, ultimately received an IEP in seventh or eighth grade.

Theme 2. Prevailing Christian Culture

A consistent and emerging theme within the focus groups centered on being Jewish in a dominant Christian public-school setting. Participants shared common stories about educating and enlightening teachers about the Jewish holidays. In some instances, their child self-advocated for their connection to Judaism and would correct those who wished them a merry Christmas or would outwardly challenge the notion of Santa. Parents felt that "there are fewer Jews, and the teachers don't quite get it." When asked what they meant by "they don't get it," they referred to the school personnel not seeing items such as chocolates of Santa, candy canes, or Christmas-related art projects as reflections of Christmas.

Parents shared experiences of class trips scheduled on high-holy Jewish holidays such as Rosh Hashanah or Yom Kippur. Participants explained they were repeatedly put in a position to request their child not feel "bothered or excluded like his life isn't easy as it is." Enlightening school staff by bringing holiday-related items or snacks remained consistent among participating parents. It was often mentioned that "Jewish parents are very involved with their kid's education." The parents did not wish to bring the religious aspect into the school but recognition of their culture. When confronted with high-holy day trips after repeated attempts to educate school personnel, one mother shared her response, "I was fairly aggravated, like, hey guys, can't you read a calendar?"

Theme 3. Jewish Supports

Most of the participants sought connections and affirmation through Jewish communities. "Generally, in public school our children are taught, if you cannot fall in line and make it easier for the teachers who are stressed by all the things who must comply with test and licensure, all the things they are, the child is the issue. In religious school, our children are valued and given so many freaking chances."

Participants of all levels of Jewish observance shared similar experiences, whether their child attended formal religious instruction, temple services, or enrolled in formal or informal Jewish recreational programs. Those whose communities had small Jewish populations sought communities they had to drive to or created their own locally. "There were no Jewish supports; the support that you had in the Jewish community was like, let's carpool to Chicago for kosher meat...there was nothing in the schools." All the parents were motivated to find a place of commonality and to have their child receive a Bar/Bat Mitzvah. "He doesn't read Hebrew, so the parsha, Haftarah, was transliterated for him and a lot of the prayers, but he led the entire service...beginning to end. He chanted; you couldn't tell that he can't read Hebrew. He was perfect. He did a speech that kind of brought down the house...we have a lot of community support here."

Outcomes from the interviews and focus group sessions indicated that public schools provide the quality of education that meets their children's needs. One participant indicated, "The teachers were amazing," and another parent expressed positive results with her son's special education, "We've seen tremendous results." Once a child's educational placement and accurate support services were secured, parents claimed to be satisfied. Autism services such as speech, occupational, and physical therapy were also satisfactory; however, parents responded with dissatisfaction to the quality of social skills groups (see Table 4.1).

While all families did express a need for public schools and providers to acknowledge the Jewish holidays and traditions, a common response from participants was that they did not expect it to be their responsibility. One parent was very satisfied with a provider's services, indicating, "we are very lucky to have found her, she's not Jewish but she recognizes that this is a thing that is significant in his life and his experience." Another expressed, "I feel like most of the educators and staff at the school try to be respectful of the fact that my kids aren't Christian." Participants provided teachers and therapeutic support professionals with Jewish holiday-related items and food and felt they were receptive. Families were primarily concerned about the needs surrounding their children's autism, above cultural sensitivity in the public domain.

Table 4.1 Respondent Results

Quality of Public-school Education	Satisfied
Quality of Autism Support Services (Speech, OT, PT)	Satisfied
Quality of Autism Support Services (Social Skills Groups)	Dissatisfied
Culturally Relevant Public-school Education	Not a priority/Satisfied
Culturally Relevant Autism Supports	Not a priority/Satisfied
Culturally Respected	Satisfied

Consistency among responses [This should be a table note provided under the table, not a part of the table]

Consistent themes emerged, reflecting key components of Jewish American parents' perceptions. The results highlighted the value that Jewish American families attributed to their children's public-school education and autism support services—apart from social skill opportunities—and their ongoing commitment to fostering Jewish identity within their homes and communities.

There is a gap in published research exploring Jewish American parents' perceptions of the cultural relevance and quality of their child's public education and autism support services. One-on-one interviews and focus group discussions generated rich outcomes. Interviews and focus group transcripts were examined for comparison and theme recognition. Anecdotal accounts and shared experiences were interpreted and synthesized. Themes emerging from the sources included public education, autism services, parent advocacy, Jewish identity, and a Christian-dominant culture. All families conveyed a solid connection to their Jewish culture, which they felt was best nourished at home and in their local communities.

Public school and autism supports were perceived as providing quality programming. Social skill groups and social skill opportunities were considered unsatisfactory. Participants identified as advocates for their children, which they reported was embedded in their culture. The voices from Jewish American parents about their experiences and perceptions of culturally responsive autism resources add to the literature that lacks the depth of cultural exploration for this population.

Parents conveyed a positive alliance with service supports and their children's public-school programming to address their child's diagnostic needs. Social skill development and profound cultural connections were missing across all formal social systems. As participants, they provided first-hand insight into the unique experiences at the intersection of their culture and the challenges of raising a child with autism. Through their voices, these parents shed light on how cultural values and practices influence their communication with service providers, schools, and community leaders. Their stories demonstrate how they internalized the need to adapt to navigate nuanced, multiplex systems to secure appropriate resources for their children while preserving their cultural identity. Their experiences highlight the importance of culturally responsive practices and reveal gaps in cultural knowledge across formal social systems. Their stories raise awareness among communities, leaders, professionals, and stakeholders about the importance of inclusivity and culturally responsive practices for Jewish families with children with autism, as well as the broader community.

This author has no conflicts of interest to declare that are relevant to the content of this chapter.

CHAPTER 5

Reflections and Significance

Abstract The significance and impact of culturally relevant social support networks are well established. Identifying the needs of Jewish American parents with a child diagnosed with autism has the potential to drive positive changes in public education, community support, and treatment practices. While parents found autism services generally relevant and helpful throughout their child's development, they frequently noted that social skill-building goals were lacking in public education programming. Cultural connections and reinforcement of an ethnic identity were found outside public schools and formal social support systems, which tend to be rooted in Christian ideologies. Many parents described a lack of acknowledgment of Jewish culture and practices, requiring them to introduce Jewish traditions and customs themselves, as these were not incorporated into the broader social systems.

Keywords Support networks · Positive change · Autism services · Ethnic identity · Lack of acknowledgment · Broader social systems

Through examining and attempting to locate published studies, no prior research on Jewish American parents' perceptions of their child with autism's public education and autism support services were found. Cultural relevance for treatment and education in autism and the rise

B. L. Raiola, *Jewish American Parents Navigating Autism Supports*,
https://doi.org/10.1007/978-3-032-29299-5_5

in autism worldwide, with little discussion in connection with Jewish American families, prompted the need for research. This case study provided a path for examining Jewish American parents' perceptions of their child's formal autism supports for enhancing service outcomes, and the development of educators, providers, and community leaders.

The significance and impact of perceptions of culturally relevant social support networks have been demonstrated. Revealing the needs of Jewish American parents with a child with autism may affect positive change in public educational, community support, and treatment practices. Parents found autism services relevant and helpful throughout their child's development. Children's goals contained a social skill-building element reportedly absent from public education system programming. Sociocultural connections and reinforcement to align with their Jewish American identity were found outside of the public school and formal social support systems based on Christian ideologies. Jewish American parents, often assumed to be part of the White dominant culture, may have a distinct culture as an ethnic and religious minority. Parents conveyed an absence of acknowledgment from their child's support systems in Jewish culture. Ethnic components, such as Jewish holidays, traditions, and food customs, were introduced by the parents and not integral to the social systems' cultures.

A summarization reflects new knowledge and research implications for implementation. Social impact through adaptive leadership was described in the context of the findings.

Jewish American parent participants with a child with autism attending or having attended public school and having received autism social supports had low to no expectations of cultural relevance in their child's education or services. Parents were satisfied with the quality of their child's education; however, delays in receiving IEPs and a lack of social skill-building opportunities or programs caused familial stress. Social and therapeutic service delivery was satisfactory, even though devoid of cultural awareness. Jewish American parents did not experience culturally relevant education or autism services. Parents were resigned to a public domain reflecting a dominant Christian culture and expected to inform teachers and providers of their child's cultural requirements, which did not negatively impact the quality of education or services.

Major themes emerged from the case study through conversational interviews and interactive focus groups. An analysis of the data reflected themes emerging as responses to interview questions included public education, autism services, parent advocacy, Jewish supports, and Christian-dominant culture (see Table 4.1). Interpretations, inferences, and conclusions aligned with and supported the findings and scope.

Parents spoke positively about their autism services; autism services received at the school, such as speech, occupational, and behavior therapies, were less effective. Services obtained from outside agencies were more qualitative and were tailored to their children's needs.

Parents reported minimal possibilities for social interactions and expressed that meaningful community opportunities through after-school groups or family events were lacking. Participants were content once their child's educational placement and accurate support services were secured. Current findings support outcomes found in studies on public education inclusion and special autism services perceived by parents as satisfactory across academics and specialized instructional supports (Al-Shams et al., 2024). While findings from autism support services were reported as satisfactory, parents expressed dissatisfaction with the quality of social skills groups as illustrated in Table 4.3 (Ma et al., 2024). Outcomes from studies supported the view that parents prioritized addressing social skills through public education for their children with autism (Ma et al., 2024). Caregivers' perceptions of educational effects may be impacted by social and cultural components relevant to their child with autism, given a severe deficit that may lead to social isolation. Participants expressed a desire for public schools and providers to acknowledge Jewish holidays and traditions, though they did not expect this need to be others' responsibility. Parents were satisfied with provider services. Caregivers devoted much of their time to seeking quality educational and social service supports that primarily addressed the needs related to their children's autism. Cultural relevance was not a primary focus, a finding consistent with other studies examining parents' priorities for their children with autism (Gholipour et al., 2022; Hamama, 2022; Sneed & Samelson, 2022).

Results from the case study highlighted parents' commitment to cultural identity, which was developed and reinforced within their Jewish homes and communities. This commitment remained distinct from the qualitative benefits associated with their children's public-school education and autism support services.

Teachers lacked awareness and preparedness for classroom inclusivity in multicultural communities globally (Sher et al., 2022). Consistent with other findings, parents educated teachers and providers about their holidays, traditions, and culture and reported that educators and service delivery providers were receptive, though inconsistent, in remembering to acknowledge Jewish holidays in their programs or school calendar (Sher et al., 2022). Jewish American parents were focused on providing their children with autism the educational and support services necessary to advance beyond any deficits associated with the diagnosis. The most religiously observant parents, whose typical children would attend Yeshivas or Jewish day schools, selected public education to ensure the best resources for school-related autism supports.

Quality-of-life criteria may be culturally specific for raising a child with autism (Bi et al., 2022; Gholipour et al., 2022) Parents from varying levels of observance, from secular to Orthodox, reported a strong connection to their Jewish identity, which emphatically contributed to a positive quality-of-life (Bi et al., 2022; Gholipour et al., 2022). Participants who attended synagogues found a sense of belonging, a community, and a strong support system for their children and their families. Parents found cultural affirmation from non-profit Jewish organizations such as Chabad, the JCC, and summer camps for Jewish children. Findings indicated that culturally relevant social supports for Jewish American parents' affirmation and quality-of-life were derived from culturally specific Jewish community networks.

Jewish American parents appear to reflect the dominant White culture; however, they may have beliefs, views, values, and unique concerns as an ethnic and religious minority (Fulton et al., 2024). While educational and autism support services were perceived to meet their intended needs, ethnic identity affirmation and cultural connections were not foundational within the public domain nor reinforced by educational or professional leaders. The literature on the training of leaders in education and healthcare conveyed a need for more professional development and formal training for working with Jewish populations (Fulton et al., 2024; Jury, 2024). Jewish American parents with a child with autism confirmed a lack of cultural awareness from educators and providers. Participants expressed the need for emotional and cultural support, which they resolved outside the public domain through local synagogues or non-profit Jewish organizations, as well as informal supports such as a circle of friends or family. Those who lived in areas where no Jewish groups existed formed their own, solidifying the assumption of the essentiality of culturally specific social supports (Bi et al., 2022; Gholipur et al., 2022). Parents' culturally specific requests were respected, except for isolated incidents that did not affect their overall perception of the quality of supports. Holidays and ethnic traditions were introduced by parents to their children's teachers and service providers and were adhered to with continued reminders or with parents supplying the items. Participants felt supported in addressing their child's deficits and educative and therapeutic needs; therefore, they were willing to provide what was needed to introduce and maintain a cultural perspective within their child's educational and service-delivery support systems.

Social support theory examines quality-of-life indicators within formal and informal network systems. Adaptive leadership theory offers a frame of reference for gauging the need for unbiased leadership to facilitate non-discriminatory, inclusive, and culturally competent programs.

Social Support Theory Applied

A social support lens aligned with an exploration of the parental perceptions of culturally relevant social structures to support Jewish American children with autism. Social support theory assumes transmission or perceived transfer of support from social networks or interpersonal connections to fulfill personal needs (Bi et al., 2022). Social capital, or resources, originated in studies of community impact and is more commonly equated with social networks (Liamputtong et al., 2022). Variables affecting individuals' health and well-being from a social support perspective include social connectedness, social capital, and social inclusion (Liamputtong et al., 2022). Research participants similarly expressed the overwhelming need to seek social networks and connections for support as Jewish Americans raising a child with autism. Parents indicated a sense of belonging found within their Jewish communities. Formal social support encompasses public education, medical, psychological, and communal networks. The literature strongly correlates improved emotional well-being plus a decline in stress and depression, with social support received by parents of children on the autism spectrum (Demšar & Bakracevic, 2023; Yan et al., 2022). Participants attributed their advocacy for their Jewish American children with autism as grounded in their Jewish values.

Jewish American families found qualitative resources and support for their child's autism educational and therapeutic requirements in the public domain. Psychological, social, cultural, and ethnic identity-related supports were found through community and informal support systems. Participants expressed no expectations from the public formal social support system networks, other than social skill opportunities, which were not adequate through the public domain.

Adaptive Leadership

An adaptive leadership approach was applied for identifying standard or commonplace leadership input to explore Jewish American parents' perceptions of the quality and cultural pertinence of therapeutic and educational support services for their child with autism (Heifetz et al., 2009). Cultural intelligence is an inherent component of adaptive leadership theory (Azevedo & Jugdev, 2022). A collective outlook that projects one's cultural perspectives onto others has been termed a cultural trap (Glover et al., 2002). Adaptive leaders challenge those they lead to adapt and assimilate in culturally variable contexts. The adaptive leadership approach promotes inclusion and acceptance in program implementation and execution, as well as safe exploration through complex exchanges (Dunn, 2020). Adaptive leadership practices provided a culturally pertinent orientation to appraise Jewish American parents' perceptions of culturally relevant autism support systems. Researchers presented a reference to identify the lack of fundamental inclusive practices in the public domain, helpful in examining structures for Jewish American families raising a child with autism (Dunn, 2020).

Jewish American parents did not experience cultural inclusivity and expressed "othering" practices, which were expected and addressed individually. Widespread discrimination in public education against ethnic groups not considered in the mainstream is perpetuated by public leaders, school administrators, principals, bureaucrats, and politicians (Pfaff et al., 2021). A commitment to secularism in the American education system, with a collective belief in Christianity, is perceived as legitimation of the American national identity (Pfaff et al., 2021). It has been proclaimed that there is a lack of Jewish cultural education, biases, and misinformation in the counseling literature (July, 2024). Scholars report Jewish identity colonization throughout clinical education and supervision among psychological professionals (Jury, 2024). The literature claims that clinicians lack the knowledge and professional development to address Jewish considerations shaped by their distinct spiritual and cultural backgrounds (Fulton et al., 2024). Adaptive leadership proponents act as group participants to foster meaningful, systemic change while steadying conflict using informal authority to reframe issues (Dunn, 2020; Heifetz et al., 2009).

The prevalent Protestant Christian ideology influences religious inclusion among American public-school leaders (Pfaff et al., 2021). Conservative Protestantism has validated American values as synonymous with American nationalism, with intolerance for minorities or atheists (Pfaff et al., 2021).

An adaptive leadership lens aligns with the case study to explore public education, medical, psychological, and communal formal support contexts relevant to Jewish American parents' perceptions of quality and culturally relevant-led education, as well as autism supports. The research indicated that adaptive leadership in the public domain to address the contextual challenges of adaptation and assimilation into diverse communities is lacking. Leaders who adopt adaptation theory rely on a range of viewpoints and microenvironments and question existing conditions and perspectives (Dunn, 2020; Heifetz et al., 2009). Diversity, multicultural, linguistic, and neurodiverse inclusion practices have taken precedence in public education and social service delivery (Giordano & Edwards, 2023; Jury, 2024; Pfaff et al., 2021). Adaptive leadership involved in contextual and systemic change, challenging the dominant, prevalent Christian-based ideologies, was absent for Jewish American parents with a child with autism in the public domain.

Adaptive leadership and social support frameworks were applicable in examining the perceptions of Jewish American parents raising a child with autism. Both approaches were relevant for assessing whether Jewish American parents' well-being and quality-of-life indicators, raising a child with autism, are perceived as recognized by formal social support leaders across domains. Jewish American parents adapted to the public school and service-delivery cultures with little expectation of their own ethnic identity being reflected in the practices. They made personal accommodations for their children across settings, consistent with findings from prior studies (Greenblatt & Koss, 2024). Leaders did not question the status quo; however, any modifications relevant to their child's ethnic accommodation were respected. Families of children with autism navigate multiple formal social support systems, which tend to lack culturally affirming services (Avery et al., 2022). In alignment with the findings, parents relied heavily on their informal supports for a sense of community, belonging, psychosocial factors contributing to their quality-of-life and well-being, and ethnic identity affirmation (Avery et al., 2022).

The study generated generalizable outcomes for comparable populations across several geographies. Further studies may pinpoint specific regions and demographics. Varying years of experience with formal support systems across the United States for children of diverse ages and autism severity levels did not impact the variability in data outcomes.

Recommendations for Further Research

Scholars reported that no studies reflecting the social perception of stigma relating to autism in Jewish communities exist (Sher et al., 2022). Within the mental health professional literature and formal training, scarce attention has been paid to understanding and working with Jewish ethno-cultural identity (Fulton et al., 2024; Jury, 2024). Research studies confirm a prevailing dominant Christian ideology equated with the notion of Americanism, impacting public education practices and policies (Greenblatt & Koss, 2024; Pfaff et al., 2021). Social service agencies serving autism populations and public education systems are prioritizing cultural and linguistic diversity policies and practices (Giordano & Edwards, 2023; Pfaff et al., 2021). Jewish Americans, however, are not included in diversity practices; rather, antisemitism and Christian nationalism reflect marginalization (Greenblatt & Koss, 2024). Jewish American parents of a child with autism report a lack of cultural affirmation in public formal social support systems and find a sense of belonging from social supports within their Jewish communities.

Current findings support the need for integrating ethnic identity affirmation and cultural connectedness in public formal, social support networks serving Jewish American children with autism. An absorption of Jewish Americans into a White Christian hegemonic social fabric is perceived as a homogeneous group (Grayson, 2023). Implicit biases contribute to anti-Semitic practices, which evoke microaggression, evidenced through dominant cultural practices foundational to American social structures, fostering a Jewish sense of otherness (Megerman, 2021). Jewish American parents described a lack of belonging, a sense of "othering," a continued need to inform educators and professionals of their cultural requirements, and shortcomings for quality social skill experiences for their children and themselves in the public domain. Opportunities for socialization for Jewish American students with autism and their parents in public schools are absent. Further research on bridging the gap between Jewish communities and public service organizations may widen opportunities for Jewish American children with autism to make more profound social connections. Linking Jewish communities and formal public social support institutions may provide less stress on Jewish American parents raising a child with autism, from continually educating teachers and professionals on their children's cultural requirements.

Recommendations emanating from the study include adaptive leaders' contribution to change within formal social support networks relevant to Jewish American parents and their children with autism. Adaptive leaders may have a systemic and contextual impact on inclusive policies and practices. Integrating Jewish American representation into public community social supports for education and social service delivery as a component of adaptive leadership practices remains an area for exploration. Neurodiverse adaptive leaders who maintain a Jewish ethno-cultural identity with influence on community public support networks are recommended for further examination.

Global Relevance

Autism spectrum disorder is a permanent condition that lasts throughout an individual's lifetime (Hamama, 2022). The need for reliance on lifelong parental support applies to approximately 85% of children with autism (de la Roche & Im-Bolter, 2024). Most individuals with autism have co-morbid conditions such as ADHD, seizure disorders, intellectual disabilities, mental illness, or anxiety (Gholipour et al., 2022). Increasing prevalence of an autism diagnosis is recognized worldwide (Gholipour et al., 2022). Research indicates parents of children with autism are among the most vulnerable and experience more stress and compromised quality-of-life than parents raising children with other developmental disabilities (Gholipour et al., 2022; Sneed & Samelson, 2022). International studies on autism emphasize the necessity of parental involvement in their child with autism's education and support services for optimal developmental outcomes (Yan et al., 2022).

Commonalities from global multicultural research findings indicated the need for culturally competent practices in service delivery and education for children with autism (Bi et al., 2022; Dira et al., 2024; Gholipour et al., 2021; Papoudi et al., 2021; Sher et al., 2022; Yan et al., 2022). Parents who perceived their formal social support systems as providing high quality, culturally relevant autism services were more engaged in their children's education and treatment worldwide (Gholipour et al., 2022). Global research outcomes suggest clinical service providers and educators require diversity training, which may yield more parental engagement (Bi et al., 2022; Dira et al., 2024; Gholipour et al., 2021; Papoudi et al., 2021; Sher et al., 2022; Yan et al., 2022). Parents raising a child with autism reported heightened stress as lifelong caregivers whose involvement in treatment and education is essential, and they remained engaged when delivery was perceived as culturally affirming.

Clinicians need to recognize the unique concerns that shape Jewish Americans' cultural identity (Fulton et al., 2024). Religious, spiritual, and ethnic dimensions may impact how an individual with autism self-identifies (Hollins et al., 2023). Ethnic identification may guide medical practices, parenting styles, and frame cultural interpretations of stigma (Hollins et al., 2023; Likhitweerawong et al., 2022; Misra et al., 2021). Parenting styles and responses may reflect a family's cultural orientation and impact a child's diagnosis, involvement, outreach, and interaction with support services (Gholipour et al., 2022; Hamama, 2022; Likhitweerawong et al., 2022). Applied behavior analysis is considered the premier therapeutic modality for working with children with autism which, according to Hollins et al. (2023), does not emphasize training in diversity, equity, and inclusion courses, particularly for marginalized populations.

Variables influencing the relationship between demographics and behavioral goal outcomes may inform culturally responsive adjustments in treatment and education for a child with autism (Jones et al., 2020). Unidentified variables relevant to cultural factors in research might affect behavioral outcomes and goals (Jones et al., 2020). The concept of cultural competency in the psychological and behavioral health arena can be extended to integrate spiritual and religious competency (Crabtree et al., 2021). Educational development and training for clinical professionals require incorporation of spiritual and religious diversity, which may affect behavioral engagement (Crabtree et al., 2021). Applied behavior analysis research traditionally lacked reporting on diversity or demographics (Hollins et al., 2023). Behavioral therapeutic practices call for culturally responsive assessment protocols, behavior plans, and culturally relevant variables in humanistic programs (Hollins et al., 2023).

Healthcare and education leaders assess and create policies for equity, diversity, and inclusion (Kuluski et al., 2021; Sunderman et al., 2020). Professional development studies in education and healthcare leadership highlight a need for additional preparation and coursework for working with Jewish populations (Fulton et al., 2024). Within social support systems, bureaucrats, politicians, and public administrators influence policies, programs, and practices (Pfaff et al., 2021). Culturally relevant training for working with Jewish American populations among educational, psychological, and behavioral professionals is scarce (Fulton et al., 2024; Jury, 2024; Greenblatt & Koss, 2024). Participant findings aligned with previous studies indicating Jewish Americans classified as White may be experiencing a sense of otherness as their distinct cultural needs are unrecognized (Grayson, 2023; Megerman, 2021).

Widespread discrimination in public education against ethnic groups not considered mainstream is reportedly perpetuated by public leaders, school administrators, principals, bureaucrats, and politicians (Pfaff et al., 2021). Adaptive leaders are needed to detect fundamental causes, motivate members to engage and collaborate, and reveal and restructure biased processes. Adaptive leaders examine cultural traps, model culturally competent leadership, and uncover unconscious behaviors to offer modifications within social structures to implement novel, relevant, and culturally applicable accommodations (Azevedo & Jugdev, 2022; Glover et al., 2002). Cultural intelligence is a dimension of adaptive leadership needed for bringing to light systemically embedded implicit bias within formal social structures.

Educational, health, and other public institutions need adaptive leadership to unearth the underlying foundations of inequitable, minoritized, and othering practices that may affect the quality of culturally responsive formal social supports (Likhitweerawong et al., 2022). Parent perceptions of their child's services correlate cultural relevance with positive wellness outcomes and satisfaction with autism programs (Jafarabadi et al., 2021). Cultural values and beliefs often shape parenting styles (Likhitweerawong et al., 2022). Jewish American parents felt the need to educate and guide educators and service providers at all leadership levels in their child's culturally specific needs. Adaptive leaders were not identified in public formal social support systems, and parents were resigned to having few expectations for culturally specific practices.

Findings indicated a lack of proactive, well-informed, culturally relevant programs and awareness of Jewish American ethno-cultural identity and practices. Literature supports the need for culturally adaptive leaders to implement systemic change. Decision-makers in the public sector, such as politicians, school administrators, and bureaucrats, would benefit from inviting leaders of Jewish American organizations to serve on their advisory boards. Jewish American families found social opportunities and social skills development lacking at formal social support organizations. Participants in the study sought ethno-cultural supports for their child with autism through their social support groups at local Jewish synagogues and non-profits, and from cultural community leaders. Faith-based organizations provided engaging youth activities, social groups, and camps for their children with autism. Data suggest the need for adaptive leaders to assess root causes in public education, healthcare, and other formal social supports, including cultural traps and biases shaped by a dominant Christian ideology (Pfaff et al., 2021).

Leaders in the behavioral and mental health arena lack cultural awareness of the needs of Jewish American families (Fulton et al., 2022; Jury, 2024). Training and educational programs for behavioral and mental health professionals have not addressed concerns unique to Jewish Americans. Research findings can impact policy change and bridge the gap between Jewish community leaders and education, healthcare, and social service systems. Leaders shape the culture of organizations and serve as models. Professional leaders can emulate, model, and adhere to self-reflection, cultural training, and inclusivity practices for Jewish American clients, where services for their children with autism are valued and essential.

Parents turned to leaders in the Jewish community and through Jewish non-profit organizations for support and affirmation not found in public education or autism support services. Jewish American parents adopted the responsibility of instilling culture and identity into their children's lives and expected to take on that role within their public-school education and autism support services. One parent engaged the leaders of the Jewish community to develop an organization for Jewish American children with autism, which later became a non-profit. Parents used their traditional foods, crafts, and artifacts to attempt to introduce and educate their children's teachers and service providers. Educators' cultural responsiveness was temporary, and parents continued to request excused absences for Jewish holidays and provide reminders to integrate Chanukkah into the winter crafts and festivities. School leaders and professionals were receptive and respectful. Sustained change to incorporate such practices into the contextual fabric was not maintained.

Behavioral and educational training programs, with input from the Jewish American community and adaptive leaders working within formal social structures, can impact social change. Discriminatory practices, microaggressions, implicit biases, and systemic antisemitism require restructuring and reframing ideologies and practices. Local workshops, Jewish community partnerships, parental advocacy groups, and interpersonal cultural exchanges may contribute to social change for Jewish American parents and their children with autism.

A qualitative case study explored Jewish American parents' perceptions of the cultural and ethnic relevance of public education and treatment received by their children with autism. Jewish American parents with a child with autism attending or having attended public school and having received autism social support had low to no expectations of cultural relevance in their child's formal social supports: education or therapeutic social services. Autism services target specific deficits and were reported to be effective.

Respondents of all Jewish denominations found quality and value in their child with autism's education and treatment. Parents who would otherwise have sent their child to Jewish day school or Yeshiva chose public school and autism supports that provided their child with the most effective autism resources as a priority above cultural relevance. Parents felt obligated to supplement public education and formal social service autism support with Jewish identity affirming materials and holiday treats.

Jewish American parents of a child with autism, whose child is or has attended public school in grades PreK-8, did not find social connections or social skill-building groups within the public education system. Parents felt respected for their cultural identity and advocated for their children's cultural needs when occasional conflicts arose at public school. Cultural connections and reinforcement for a Jewish American ethno-cultural identity were found outside of the public school and autism service arena, where families maintained a separate circle of informal supports.

Jewish American parents expressed the need to advocate for their child with autism as a priority and then to ensure cultural awareness across contexts where they received education and therapeutic support. Integrating educational and treatment support found in the public domain, along with Jewish cultural connectedness, is a further area for exploration. Educators, treatment professionals, public administrators, and leaders need to make profound systemic changes to bridge the gap and recognize the prospective social isolation of Jewish American children and other marginalized, non-Christian students with autism who are unable to make social and culturally relevant connections in their daily formal social support systems based on Christian ideologies and practices. By centering the voices of Jewish American parents navigating autism supports, this study contributes to research and recommendations grounded in authentic, culturally contextualized experiences, resulting in a more impactful, understanding support for families.

As the principal researcher conducting this qualitative study on Jewish American parents navigating autism supports, I recognize that my own social position, background, and experiences inevitably shape my approach to this research. I am aware that factors such as my cultural identity, academic training, personal beliefs, and previous interactions within both Jewish and autism communities influence the questions I ask, the way I interpret data, and the relationships I build with participants.

I acknowledge that I bring both knowledge and assumptions to this work. My own perspective—whether as an insider, outsider, or somewhere in between with respect to the Jewish community or the experience of interacting with those parenting a child with autism—can inform my sensitivity to certain issues while potentially blinding me to others. I strived to maintain reflexivity throughout the research process by continually examining how my positionality may affect data collection, analysis, and interpretation. I have been committed to fostering an open, respectful environment during interviews and to listening deeply to participants' lived experiences, recognizing that their voices are central to this study.

To mitigate the influence of my biases, I engaged in ongoing self-reflection and sought feedback from peers and community stakeholders. By being transparent about my social position and its possible impact, I aim to enhance the trustworthiness and authenticity of the research findings. My goal is to honor the complexity and diversity of Jewish American parents' experiences as they navigate autism supports, while acknowledging the limitations of my own perspective.

This author has no conflicts of interest to declare that are relevant to the content of this chapter.

References

Al-Shams, F., Hossain, S., Sakib, A. S., Arjuman, H., Chakraborty, S. M., & Afridi, S. (2024). Perspectives among parents of children with autism on inclusive education. *Journal of Medical and Clinical Case Reports, 1*(10), 1–6. https://doi.org/10.61615/JMCCR/2024/SEPT027140920

Avery, K., van Rhijn, T., & Maich, K. (2022). Understanding the role of formal and informal support resources for parent of children with autism spectrum disorder. *Canadian Journal of Family and Youth, 14*(3), 32–51. https://ejournals.library.ualberta.ca/index/php/cify

Azevedo, A., & Jugdev, K. (2022). Applying cultural intelligence to develop adaptive leadership. *Organization Development Journal, 40*(4), 56–70. https://research.ebsco.com/linkprocessor/plink?id=52a7db82-3588-3df3-81badfbc7ce30a90

Bi, X., He, H., Lin, H., & Fan, X. (2022). Influence of social support network and perceived social support on the subjective well-being of mothers of children with autism spectrum disorder. *Frontiers in Psychology, 13*. https://doi.org/10.3389/fpsyg.2022.835110

Crabtree, S. A., Bell, C. A., Rupert, D. A., Sandage, S. J., Devor, N. G., & Stavros, G. (2021). Humility, differentiation of self, and clinical training in spiritual and religious competence. *Journal of Spirituality in Mental Health, 23*(4), 342–362. https://doi.org/10.1080/19349637.2020.1737627

de la Roche, L., & Im-Bolter, N. (2024). A qualitative analysis of parent's perceptions of available social support systems. *Discover Psychology, 4*(1), 1–7. https://doi.org/10.1007/s44202-024-00293-5

Demšar, A., & Bakracevic, K. (2023). Depression, anxiety, stress, and coping mechanisms among parents of children with autism spectrum disorder. *International Journal of Disability, Development and Education, 70*(6), 994–1007. https://doi.org/10.1080/1034912X.2021.1947474

Dira, P. M. M., Machailo, R. J., & Scholtz, S. (2024). Caregivers' voices: From the world of autism spectrum disorder. *Curationis, 47*(1), 1–11. https://doi.org/10.4102/curationis.v47i1.2519

Dunn, R. (2020). Adaptive leadership: Leading through complexity. *International Studies in Educational Administration, 48*(1), 31–38. http://hdl.handle.net/11343/258917

Fulton, C. L., Melamed, L., & Lambert, A. (2024). Ethno-religious engagement, minority experiences, and strengthening American Jewish identity. *Journal of Mental Health Counseling, 46*(3), 223–258. https://doi.org/10.17744/mehc.46.3.03

Gholipour, K., Ghiasi, A., Shahrokhi, H., Dadashi, Z., Javanmard, S., Tabatabaei, S. H., & Iezadi, S. (2022). Perceptions of the professionals and parents of children with autism spectrum disorders about autism services; a qualitative study. *Journal of Autism and Developmental Disorders, 53*(1), 96–109. https://doi.org/10.1007/s10803-021-05388-9

Giordano, G., & Edwards, J. (2023). *Enhancing cultural responsiveness in social service agencies, OPRE Report # 2023-338*. Prepared by Insight Policy Research. U.S. Department of Health and Human Services.

Glover, J., Friedman, H., & Jones, G. (2002). Adaptive leadership: When change is not enough (part two). *Organization Development Journal,*

20(4), 18–38. https://www.proquest.com/scholarly-journals/adaptive-leadership-part-two-four-principles/docview/197987737/se-2

Grayson, M. L. (2023). Assimilation/appropriation: What Jewish discourses in rhetoric, composition, and writing studies tell us about the limitations of inclusion. *College Composition and Communication, 75*(1), 56–74. https://www.proquest.com/scholarly-journals/assimilation-appropriation-what-jewish-discourses/docview/2897296853/se-2

Greenblatt, D., & Koss, M. D. (2024). Antisemitism as an integral part of anti-bias educational policies and practices. *Journal for Multicultural Education, 18*(4), 385–395. https://doi.org/10.1108/JME-08-2023-0072

Hamama, L. (2022). Perceived social support, normalization, and subjective well-being among family members of a child with autism spectrum disorder. *Journal of Autism and Developmental Disorders*. https://doi.org/10.1007/s10803-022-05857-9

Heifetz, R., Grashow, A., & Linsky, M. (2009). *The practice of adaptive leadership: Tools and tactics for changing your organization and the world*. Harvard Business School Publishing. https://doi.org/10.1111/j.1744-6570.2009.01168_4.x

Hollins, N. A., Morris, C., & Li, A. (2023). Integrating diversity, equity, and inclusion readings within coursework: Suggestions for instructors teaching behavior analysis. *Behavior Analysis in Practice*. https://doi.org/10.1007/s40617-023-00781-5

Jafarabadi, M.A., Gholipour, K., Shahrokhi, H., Malek, A., Ghiasi, A., Pourasghari, H. & Iezadi, S. (2021). Disparities in the quality of and access to services in children with autism spectrum disorders: a structural equation modeling. *Archives of Public Health, 79*(1), 1–11. https://doi.org/10.1186/s13690-021-00577-5

Jones, S. H., St Peter, C. C., & Ruckle, M. M. (2020). Reporting of demographic variables in the journal of applied behavior analysis. *Journal of Applied Behavior Analysis, 53*(3), 1304–1315. https://doi.org/10.1002/jaba.722

Jury, R. T. (2024). Cultural considerations when working with Jewish students and supervisees. *The Clinical Supervisor, 1–23*. https://doi.org/10.1080/07325223.2024.2413060

Kuluski, K., Reid, R. J., & Baker, G. R. (2021). Applying the principles of adaptive leadership to person-centered care for people with complex care needs. *Health Expectations, 24*(2), 175–181. https://doi.org/10.1111/hex.13174

Liamputtong, P., Rice, Z. S., & Suwankhong, D. (2022). Social capital and social inclusion. In P. Liamputtong (Ed.), *Handbook of social inclusion* (pp. 43–57). Springer. https://doi.org/10.1007/978-3-030-89594-5_3

Likhitweerawong, N., Boonchooduang, N., & Louthrenoo, O. (2022). Parenting styles, parental stress, and quality of life among caregivers of Thai children with autism. *International Journal of Disability, Development &*

Education, 69(6), 2094–2107. https://doi.org/10.1080/1034912X.2020.1837354

Ma, Z., Fu, W., Gu, P., Siting, H., Liujing, Y., & Zhou, W. (2024). Parental perception of the importance of friendship and other educational outcomes in children with autism spectrum disorder in China. *Journal of Autism & Developmental Disorders, 54*(5), 2012–2025. https://doi.org/10.1007/s10803-023-05954-3

Megerman, S. (2021). Voices across the spectrum breaking down "othering" within law librarianship. *American Association of Law Libraries (AALL) Spectrum, 26*(2), 38–40. https://research.ebsco.com/linkprocessor/plink?id=0f5d74d6-990b-3193-a3d8-9176340a7aad

Misra, S., Jackson, V. W., Chong, J., Choe, K., Tay, C., Wong, J., & Yang, L. H. (2021). A systematic review of cultural aspects of stigma and mental illness among racial and ethnic minority groups in the United States: Implications for interventions. *American Journal of Community Psychology, 68*(3/4), 486–512. https://doi.org/10.1002/ajcp.12516

Papoudi, D., Jørgensen, C. R., Guldberg, K., & Meadan, H. (2021). Perceptions, experiences, and needs of parents of culturally and linguistically diverse children with autism: A scoping review. *Review Journal of Autism and Developmental Disorders, 8*(2), 195–212. https://doi.org/10.1007/s40489-020-00212-1

Pfaff, S., Crabtree, C., Kern, H. L., & Holbein, J. B. (2021). Do street-level bureaucrats discriminate based on religion? A large-scale correspondence experiment among American public school principals. *Public Administration Review, 81*(2), 244–259. https://doi.org/10.1111/puar.13235

Sher, D. A., Gibson, J. L., & Sher, H. E. (2022). "We've come a very, very, long way" overcoming stigma of autism: An interpretative phenomenological analysis within the UK Jewish community. *Autism: The International Journal of Research & Practice, 26*(8), 2066–2083. https://doi.org/10.1177/13623613221075099

Sneed, L., & Samelson, D. (2022). Effectiveness of parent-led applied behavior analysis at improving outcomes for parents of autistic children. *Journal of Social, Behavioral & Health Sciences, 16*(1), 160–177. https://doi.org/10.5590/JSBHS.2022.16.1.12

Sunderman, H. M., Headrick, J., & McCain, K. (2020). Addressing complex issues and crises in higher education with an adaptive leadership framework. *Change, 52*(6), 22–29. https://doi.org/10.1080/00091383.2020.1839322

Yan, T., Hou, Y., & Deng, M. (2022). The direct, indirect, and buffering effect of social support on parental involvement among Chinese parents of children with autism spectrum disorders. *Journal of Autism and Developmental Disorders, 52*(7), 2911–2923. https://doi.org/10.1007/s10803-021-05170-x

Index

B. L. Raiola, *Jewish American Parents Navigating Autism Supports*,
https://doi.org/10.1007/978-3-032-29299-5

GPSR Compliance
The European Union's (EU) General Product Safety Regulation (GPSR) is a set of rules that requires consumer products to be safe and our obligations to ensure this.

If you have any concerns about our products, you can contact us on

ProductSafety@springernature.com

In case Publisher is established outside the EU, the EU authorized representative is:

Springer Nature Customer Service Center GmbH
Europaplatz 3
69115 Heidelberg, Germany

www.ingramcontent.com/pod-product-compliance
Ingram Content Group UK Ltd.
Pitfield, Milton Keynes, MK11 3LW, UK
UKHW040342180926
475648UK00001B/2
* 9 7 8 3 0 3 2 2 9 2 9 8 8 *